Published by:
Association of Reflexologists Ltd
5-6 Fore Street
Taunton
Somerset
TA1 1HX

+44 (0)1823 351010
www.aor.org.uk

ISBN: 978-0-9933909-0-6

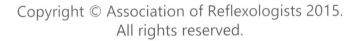

Contents

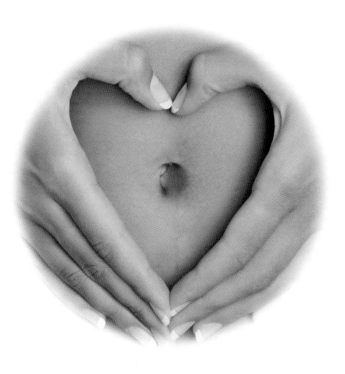

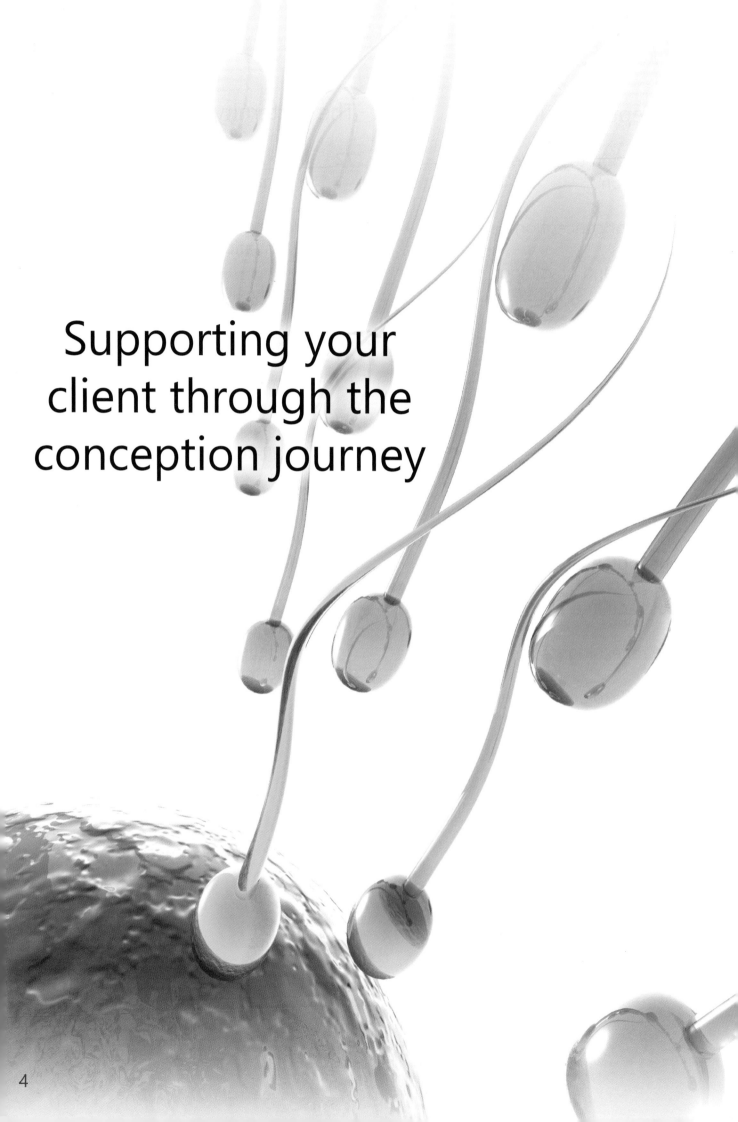

Supporting your client through the conception journey

Introduction to *reflexology through the conception journey*

This section is designed to impart information on a complicated area of the human body. If you have clients who have been trying to conceive, you need to understand what they are going through, both physically and emotionally, and that is what we hope you will take away from this booklet.

However, we do start with a word of caution: as you are aware, we are limited in what we can claim in our advertising and marketing (ASA recommendations). You must use your gained knowledge carefully and with sensitivity and do not make major claims on the back of this knowledge. We would suggest that you say you have 'completed further studies in the area of conception', or 'have a deeper understanding of this area', which after reading this book will be true. The area of conception is definitely one where we as therapists need to be ultra aware of the effects on the body of stress and the emotions. Stress is incredibly important in fertility and therefore is very linked to conception - so remember; we can say that reflexology helps relax, improves mood, aids sleep, helps relieve tension and improves a sense of wellbeing which, in theory, can help improve a couple's chance of conceiving.

We also put this book together to help dispel some of the myths regarding this area. You can treat most of the time but there are time points when it is best for all that you don't. We hope to calm some of the fears about the question of when to treat and when not and to promote confidence.

We hope you come out at the end with more knowledge than you started with!

Sally Earlam FMAR and Tracey Smith FMAR

P.S. The reading of this book and any further follow up reading gains you CPD points - don't forget to log one point for every hour you spend reading about conception and related topics.

Fertility or conception?

The medical term for problems with getting pregnant is infertility. But is this in fact a misnomer? Fertility is the meeting of the egg and the sperm from two individuals and their joining together to product a new mix of DNA. But it does not mean the woman becomes pregnant, this only occurs at the implantation stage. Some couples may be very fertile but just never have the implantation stage succeed. Some may have perfect implantation mechanisms but never have a baby because fertilisation fails every time.

In actuality having a baby is not about fertility or implantation but is the interconnection of the two systems to allow for conception. As in everything in life – it is about balance.

Anatomy and physiology of the
reproductive system

Female

The female reproductive system allows for the production of eggs, a place for the egg to attach if fertilised and a place for the baby to grow. The reproductive organs also include the breasts to feed the baby, but these are not going to be discussed here as they are not related to conception.

Ovary – these are the production centres of the eggs. A female baby is born with all the eggs she will ever have; this is known as the ovarian reserve and as the female matures, so do the eggs. At puberty they begin to release approximately one per month, although this may vary with the individual. Every month, 20 or so follicles are stimulated and begin to mature to produce an egg; usually only one fully matured egg will be released. Production of oestrogen, progesterone and testosterone comes from the ovaries.

Fallopian tube – This is the connecting tube from the ovary to the uterus. They are also rather old-fashionedly known as salpinges (hence the hysteriosalpingogram test). At the ovary end there is a fringe of tissue called the fimbriae that sweeps over the ovary and collects the eggs released. Propelled by the movement of cilia, the eggs then pass down the tube into the uterus where fertilisation can take place.

Fallopian Tube   Uterus   Fundus   Uterine Tube

Fimbriae   Ovary

Endometrium

Myometrium

Vagina

Cervix

Uterus – this is a muscular organ lined with endometrial cells that undergoes changes through the menstrual cycle under the effect of the reproductive hormones – see page 8. It is where the embryo will implant and where the placenta integrates itself. The uterus expands to cope with the size of the baby and shrinks back again after birth.

Cervix – this is a cylinder shaped ring of tissue connecting the uterus to the vagina. The cervix produces mucus throughout the month that changes to be for or against sperm depending on the time of the month. It has a hole in the centre which allows for the passage of menstrual blood and the baby in one direction and sperm in the opposite direction. During pregnancy the cervix helps to hold the baby in place and then in labour it dilates greatly to allow the baby to pass through it. The extent of the dilation indicates the stage of labour.

http://women.webmd.com/picture-of-the-cervix

Vagina – muscular passage that connects the uterus to the outside.

Male

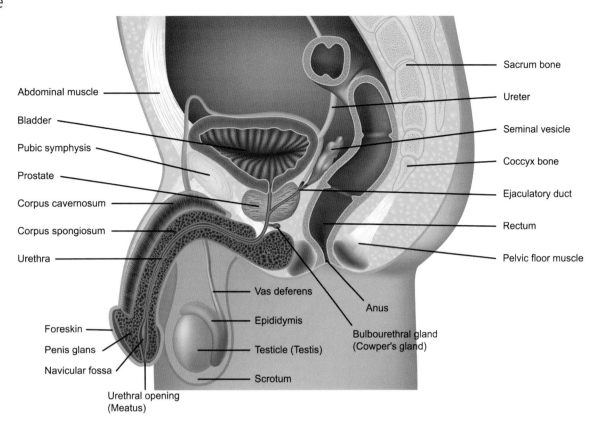

Abdominal muscle
Bladder
Pubic symphysis
Prostate
Corpus cavernosum
Corpus spongiosum
Urethra

Foreskin
Penis glans
Navicular fossa
Urethral opening (Meatus)

Vas deferens
Epididymis
Testicle (Testis)
Scrotum

Anus
Bulbourethral gland (Cowper's gland)

Sacrum bone
Ureter
Seminal vesicle
Coccyx bone
Ejaculatory duct
Rectum
Pelvic floor muscle

Testes – these are egg shaped organs where the main functions are to produce sperm and androgens which include testosterone. While they are in the testes, the sperm are very immature and would not fertilise an egg. Most cells in the human body have two pairs of chromosomes; however, gametes can only have one set as they have to join with another cell to evolve into a new individual with mixed DNA. Therefore, during the process of maturation, the sperm have to reduce the number of chromosomes (or diplody) to one set. This happens during the sperm's time in the testes; however, when they leave they are still not able to move and so are squeezed out of the testes to the next process.

The whole process of sperm production takes 64 days and is very sensitive to changes in temperature, hormones and illness. In men, the optimal temperature is two degrees below body temperature; therefore periods where the body has a raised temperature (for example a fever) can have a negative effect on sperm quality.

The mature but not yet motile sperm are squeezed into the epididymis, where they gain motility and the ability to fertilise under the action of epididymal-specific and androgen-dependent secretory proteins. Vitamin D also seems to be important in the motility of sperm. http://www.ncbi.nlm.nih.gov/pubmed/6360113

http://www.ncbi.nlm.nih.gov/pubmed/21427118

Vas Deferens – the tube leading from the epididymis to the urethra via the prostate and seminal vesicles. The newly motile sperm are not expected to do any work here as they are moved by peristaltic motion up the vas deferens to the urethra. The vas deferens is the tube that is cut or tied in a vasectomy.

Prostate – this 'slightly larger than a walnut' sized organ produces alkaline secretions that make up about 20% of the semen.

Seminal vesicles – these two glands also produce secretions, but this time the secretions contain prostaglandins, energy enabling fructose and other ions. The prostaglandins are thought to aid fertilisation by preparing the cervix to become more receptive to sperm. This is about 60% of the total semen. http://www.britannica.com/EBchecked/topic/534058/seminal-vesicle

Bladder – the bladder holds urine until it is expelled.

Urethra – the urethra travels down the penis and carries both urine and sperm. Both fluids have to flow past the prostate, the enlargement of which can cause problems with both systems.

Penis – this contains erectile tissue, allowing for intercourse to take place.

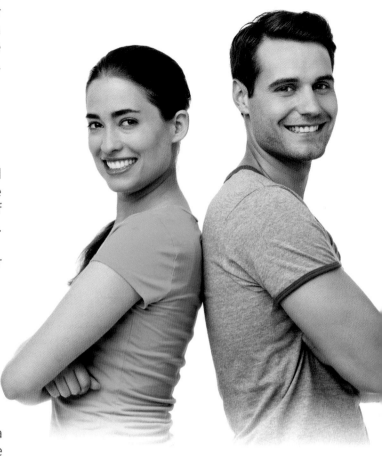

Female Hormones

The total picture of hormones in the non-pregnant and pregnant female is complicated, but nevertheless needs to be understood.

Gonadotrophin releasing hormone (GnRH) – this is a neuropeptide that is released in both sexes from the hypothalamus. It acts on the pituitary, causing the release of the gonadotrophins FSH and LH, which act in both males and females on different cells. In females, the release of GnRH is by pulses from the hypothalamus, which is dependent on the variability of the menstrual cycle, while in males it is pulse released at a constant frequency.

Follicle stimulating hormone (FSH) – this is produced by the pituitary and causes the young, small follicles to mature. Higher levels of oestrogen just before ovulation turn the production of FSH off.

Luteinising hormone (LH) – this is produced by the pituitary and causes the egg to release. Levels drop quickly afterwards.

Oestrogen - This is produced by the ovary and has a positive effect on the pituitary, increasing production of luteinising hormone (LH); conversely, the same high levels of oestrogen reduce the production of Follicle Stimulating hormone (FSH). This turns off egg maturation but turns on the egg release process.

Progesterone – this is produced by the ovary and slowly increases over the second half of the cycle. Its job is to maintain the endometrium. If a fertilised embryo implants, the endometrium remains thick and spongy ready for placental growth. If there is no implantation, the progesterone concentration drops quickly, causing the endometrium to slough off; this results in a period.

Process of ovulation

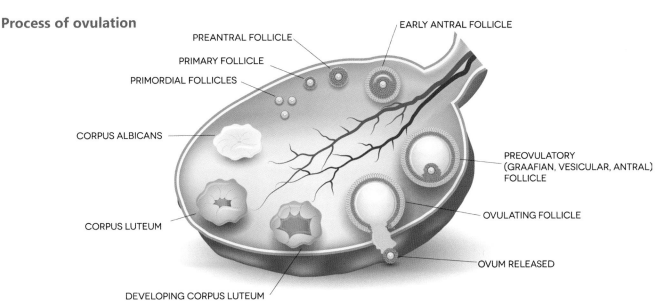

Follicles – these mature from primordial follicles over 13 menstrual cycles or 375 days to rupture and release the egg. The first part of the maturation happens under the action of androgens produced by the surrounding thecal cells, while the latter stages of follicle maturation are promoted by FSH and LH.

Corpus luteum – this is what is left of the follicle after the egg has been released. LH induces the corpus luteum to produce progesterone which promotes and maintains the endometrium. If there is no fertilisation around 22 days after egg release, the corpus luteum starts to decline to become a corpus albicans, which is a mass of fibrous scar tissue. The oestrogen and progesterone levels also decline, allowing for an increase in FSH to bring about the maturation of the follicles for the next cycle. As the progesterone drops, it causes the endometrium to fail and menstruation starts.

Human Chorionic Gonadotrophin (HCG)

This is a hormone produced by the fertilisation and subsequent implantation of the embryo at around day 9 post fertilisation. It is produced by cells originating from the trophoblast cells and it prevents the corpus luteum from degrading, thus allowing the production of progesterone to continue. This keeps the endometrium active and no period results.

http://www.gfmer.ch/Presentations_En/Menstrual_cycle/Menstrual_cycle_Bischof.htm

http://en.wikipedia.org/wiki/Corpus_luteum

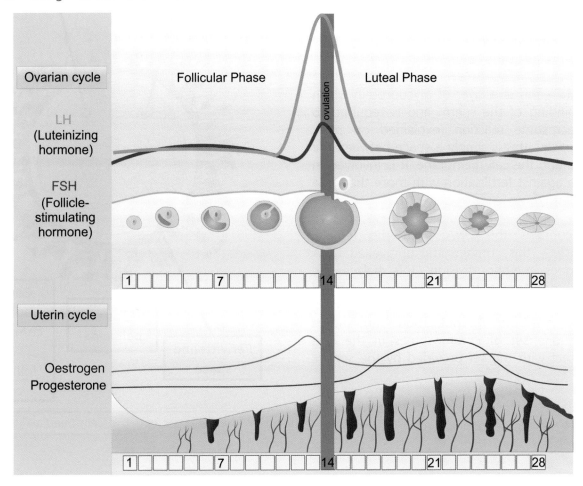

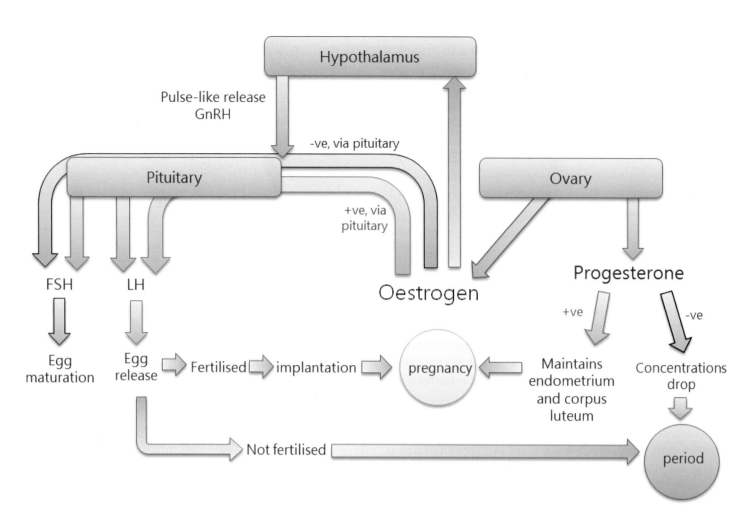

Structure of an egg

The corona radiata – this comprises of follicular cells and does two important jobs: the cells protect the egg in its journey from the follicle to the uterus and they provide vital proteins to the cell.

Zona pellucida – this is a layer of glycoprotein which enables the binding of the sperm and is required to initiate the acrosome reaction (explained on p11). Perivitteline space – this is simply a space between the zona pellucida and the cell membrane. It is involved in the protection against fertilisation with more than one sperm (polyspermy).

Nucleus – contains the DNA from the female. Germinal vesicle – this contains the unravelled DNA which undergoes meiotic division; this halves the number of chromosomes from 2 sets (the normal adult cell number or diploid) to one set (haploid). The second set goes into the polar body (not shown here), leaving one set of chromosomes in the egg ready to interact with the set provided by the sperm.

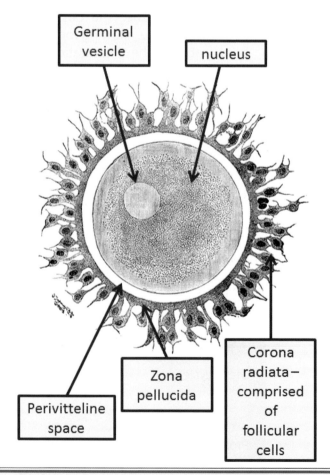

https://en.wikipedia.org/wiki/Egg_cell#/media/File:Gray3.png

Structure of sperm

Head - The head consists of a membrane surrounding the acrosome and the nucleus containing DNA. The acrosome is an enzyme pocket which releases the enzymes when the membrane of the head binds to the outer surface of the egg, allowing the nucleus DNA to float freely into the egg.

Midpiece - This is the 'battery' for the sperm and it contains all the power to keep the sperm moving until it reaches the egg.

Tail - This is the element of the sperm that allows it to move, the flicking backwards and forwards causes forwards propulsion.

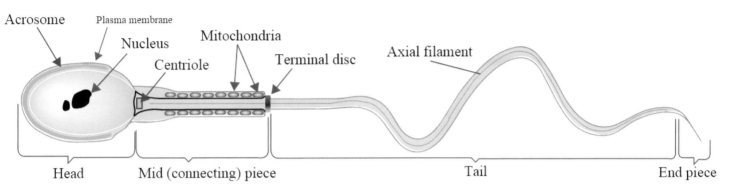

http://en.wikipedia.org/wiki/File:Complete_diagram_of_a_human_spermatozoa_en.svg

Fertilisation

A single sperm enters the egg; this has to be only a single sperm because if multiple sperm (polyspermy) enter the egg then there will be too many chromosomes and the embryo dies early. Sperm have to undergo several changes before they are capable of fertilisation, which are collectively called capacitation. Seminal plasma proteins are removed and plasma membrane lipids and proteins are reorganized. Capacitation also probably breaks down the external proteins ready for the acrosome reaction. The sperm binds to the zona pellucida of the egg by interaction with the proteins in the zona pellucida and then the acrosome reaction takes place. The acrosome is a pocket of enzymes that allows the head of the sperm to melt through the zona pellucida and the egg wall which, together with the beating of the sperm tail, deposits the sperm DNA inside the egg. Binding of the sperm proteins with the zona pellucida triggers a reaction, causing it to harden and a destruction of the surface sperm receptors. This prevents any further sperm entering the egg, thus preventing polyspermy.

Once the sperm has entered the egg, there are two free floating, unravelled bundles of DNA inside the nuclear membrane, each of which equate to half the number of chromosomes in a normal cell.

These quickly become bound by a fresh nuclear membrane to form two pronuclei which naturally float towards each other and then become joined together. The DNA fuses and new chromosomes are formed with a mixture of DNA from the mother and the father.

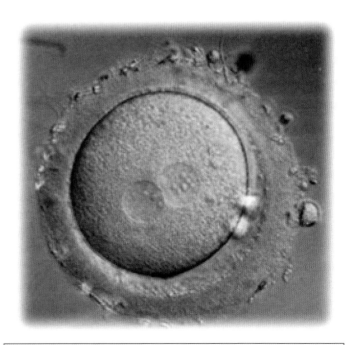

Early embryo showing pronuclei
courtesy of Dr P Renwick, Centre for Preimplantation
Genetic Diagnosis, Guy's Hospital, London UK

Pronuclei 1-cell stage	Two-cell stage	Four-cell stage	Eight-cell stage

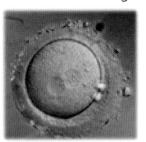  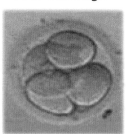 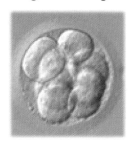

10-12 cell stage	Morula stage	Blastocyst stage	Hatching blastocyst stage

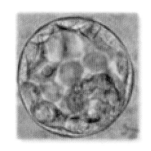 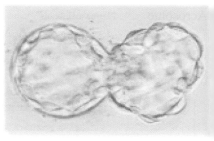

Day 1 post fertilisation - the single cell cleaves (splits) into two cells. This is the beginning of new life. It is also the most likely point where the embryos can arrest or stop growing.

Day 2 - the cells split to four and then again to eight.

Day 3 - the eight cells split again to 16 and then 32; at this point it's called a morula

Day 4 - the morula compacts into a ball of cells so that each individual cell cannot be distinguished.

Day 5 – 6 - the cells separate into two different cell layers with a visible cavity; the layer on the inside is going to be the baby and the other on the outside will be the placenta. This is called a blastocyst. At this point the embryo is still floating free in the fallopian tube/uterus.

Day 6-7 - Hatching and Implantation

The zona pellucida around the egg that was protective now becomes constraining, so enzymes start to break down the protein which allows the embryo to squeeze its way out. Next, the cells on the surface of the blastocyst change to become enlarged and sticky (trophoblast cells). The endometrium is also undergoing changes, producing decidual cells and pinopodes – these cells reduce the volume of fluid in the uterus, allowing the embryo to be closer to the walls of the uterus and therefore more likely to stick. The trophoblast cells change to trophoblast giant cells which then escape from the embryo and start to invade into the surface of the endometrium, resulting in attachment

and eventually the setting up of a circulatory system that becomes the placenta. During this part of the pregnancy, it is possible that there may be slight breakthrough bleeding.

Human chorionic gonadotrophin (HCG) is produced by the invading cells from the embryo; this is what is measured in a pregnancy test and is what defines pregnancy. There is a required time frame for the release of this hormone, which is about 14 days after egg collection in assisted cycles or ovulation in non assisted cycles.

If implantation doesn't succeed and the pregnancy test is negative, then progesterone levels drop, the endometrium sloughs off and the woman has a period.

If there is a positive pregnancy test the GP should be informed,they will arrange an antenatal appointment and probably an ultrasound scan for around the 12 week mark.

If the pregnancy has been through assisted conception they will often arrange an extra 6 week scan to check for a heartbeat and for multiple pregnancies. After the 12 week scan an IVF pregnancy will be transferred over to normal antenatal care.

After a positive cardiac scan, the next milestone is the standard 12 week scan and this is where an IVF pregnancy is then transferred over to normal antenatal care.

http://www.vivo.colostate.edu/hbooks/pathphys/reprod/fert/fert.html

Determining *the day of ovulation*

Remember that the best advice for couples who are trying to conceive is that they should try and have sexual intercourse every 2-3 days, regardless of where the woman is in her cycle. This is based on the fact that an ovum will only survive for about 12-24 hours after it is released; the ovum needs to be fertilised by a sperm within this time or else it will begin to break down. Sperm, however, can live for up to seven days inside a woman's body, so if the couple are having regular intercourse then there should be sperm present in the fallopian tube ready to meet the egg, regardless of when the woman actually ovulates.

In summary, this means that women are potentially fertile for up to 6 days before they ovulate and for only one day after they ovulate.

The NICE guidelines (see page 36 for more information on NICE) also state:

"People who are concerned about their fertility should be informed that vaginal sexual intercourse every 2 to 3 days optimises the chance of pregnancy"

National Institute for Health and Care Excellence (2013) Adapted from CG 156 Fertility: assessment and treatment for people with fertility problems. Manchester: NICE. Available from www.nice.org.uk/CG156. Reproduced with permission.

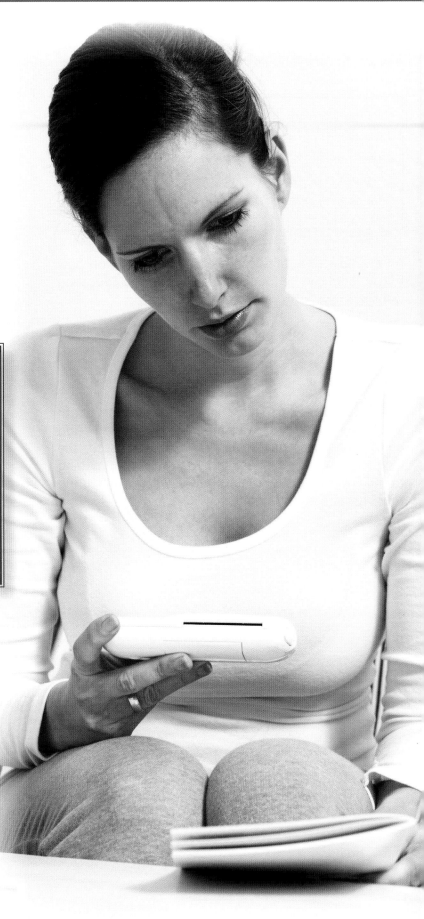

It is important to reinforce this point of view to clients, yet you will frequently see in clients who have been trying to conceive for a while that they are either worried that they are not ovulating, or that they feel they want to know when they are ovulating so they can make a concerted effort to have sexual intercourse around this time. Although the latter is not recommended, they may still feel they want to know. It is, however, very important for the couple to remember (and you may wish to remind them) that lovemaking should be enjoyed to nurture a relationship; it is not just for the sole function of making babies!

Another helpful piece of advice might be for the couple not to have sexual intercourse more than once a day as sperm may become immature and less motile.

Natural fertility awareness

There are signs in the body that help identify when ovulation is taking place. To maximize the accuracy of these calculations, there are three main methods that should be used in combination. As the length of a menstrual cycle and day of ovulation can vary over time, to ensure the calculations are as accurate as possible it is recommended that the details below are charted over the course of six months. In the meantime, you can again reinforce that they should try and have regular intercourse.

> The details to chart are:
>
> 1. Calculations of where they are in their menstrual cycle
> 2. daily readings of body temperature
> 3. secretions of mucus from the cervix
>
> Optionally, one could also chart the position of cervix as well.

An example of fertility charts and information on how to use them can be found at the Fertility and Education website: www.fertilityet.org.uk/charts.html.

There are also apps available to download onto smart phones that allow women to keep records.

1. Menstrual cycle

The first information that should be charted is the length of the menstrual cycle with the first day of the period being charted as day 1. As previously discussed, the length of a woman's menstrual cycle can vary - anything from 24 to 35 days is common with ovulation occurring roughly half way through the cycle.

2. Basal body temperature

The second sign that should be charted is body temperature; this method is based on the fact that there is a small rise in body temperature after ovulation takes place.

As the rise in temperature is small; usually around 0.2C (0.4F) either a digital thermometer or a thermometer specifically designed to be used for natural family planning needs to be used; these are available from pharmacies.

The temperature method involves:

- Taking the temperature every morning before getting out of bed, this should be done before eating, drinking or smoking and ideally at the same time every morning.
  - ➤ Before ovulation the temperature remains low.
  - ➤ After ovulation the temperature rises and will remain high until the next period begins.
  - ➤ After 3 days of a raised temperature the fertile period for that month is over.

- There are other factors that can cause a rise in temperature such as:
  - Taking it at different times;
  - Being ill, having a fever, a migraine etc.
  - A hang-over
  - A late night or a disturbed night's sleep.
  - Jet lag

If a rise occurs at an unusual time, any possible explanation should be recorded.

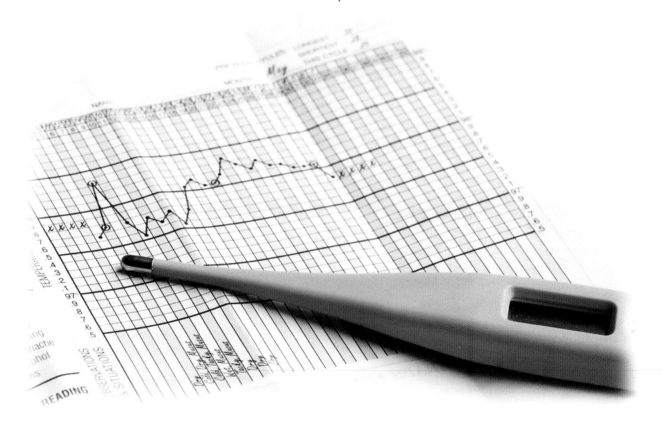

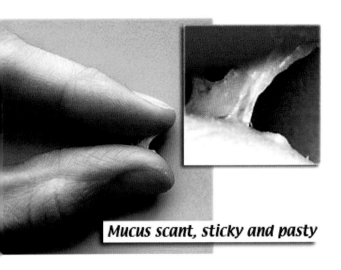

Mucus scant, sticky and pasty

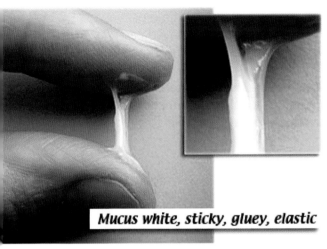

Mucus white, sticky, gluey, elastic

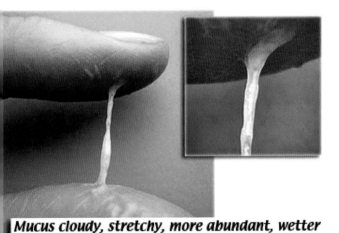

Mucus cloudy, stretchy, more abundant, wetter

Mucus clear, stretchy, profuse, slippery, wet

3. Cervical secretions

There is also a change in the consistency and amount of the mucus secreted from the cervix during different times in the menstrual cycle that needs to be charted. One advantage of this method is that the changes occur as ovulation approaches which gives the women fore-warning that her fertile period is approaching, whereas the temperature only increases after ovulation.

Cervical secretions can be checked by gently placing the middle finger into the vagina or wiping over the vulva with toilet tissue and observing what is on the paper. The changes that will occur throughout the cycle are listed below, describing what happens after the period finishes:

- For the first few days after the period, the vagina will be dry and little or no secretions will be felt.

- Then mucous will become present but it will be scant, sticky and pasty.

- The amount of cervical secretions continues to increase, and will begin to appear to be cloudy, white and sticky.

- As ovulation approaches, the amount of secretions will continue to increase until it becomes more profuse, slippery, clear and stretchy between the fingers – it is often referred to as egg white consistency at this stage; ovulation is now very close and the secretions are perfect for sperm to be able to swim in. This is the most fertile period.

- Ovulation occurs on the last day of the egg white consistency secretions; after ovulation, the secretions will again begin to dry up.

Pictures used with kind permission from Colleen Norman. http://www.fertilityet.org.uk/

Optional: Shape and position of the cervix

This is another method that some women may use to help assess their day of ovulation as the shape and position of the cervix changes throughout the menstrual cycle. This is not something that all women will be comfortable to do as it does involve internal examination. We are not suggesting that you need to discuss this method with clients; the 3 changes previously discussed should be adequate to map ovulation. But you should be aware of it in case a client is using this method and wishes to discuss it with you.

How to examine the cervix – advise clients to:

- Start when menstrual bleeding has stopped.
- Check it at the same time each day; it is easiest to do at the end of each day as the cervix is always lower in the evenings.
- The cervix can be felt either squatting, sitting on the toilet, or with one foot raised on a stool.
- Gently insert one finger (or two) high into the vagina, as you would insert a tampon.
- Check the position, shape and opening of the cervix.

Before ovulation, the cervix will feel:

FIRM - like the tip of the nose
LOW - easy to reach
CLOSED
DRY

Approaching ovulation, the cervix will feel:

SOFT - like the chin
HIGH - harder to reach
OPEN
WET

After ovulation, the cervix will feel:

FIRM - like the tip of the nose
LOW - easy to reach
CLOSED
DRY

Ovulation predictor kits (OPK)

Generally ovulation kits are thought to be the most accurate way of determining when the woman's most fertile time is each month. However this can become quite expensive as it may need on average 5 - 7 tests per month. There are a number of OPK's available; the most widely available are kits that test a urine sample for levels of luteinizing hormone (LH). A day or two before ovulation, the level of LH dramatically increases and this surge of LH is a reliable indicator that the woman is heading into her most fertile period.

As a general guide, if a woman takes the length of her normal cycle, divides this in half and then subtracts 3-4 days – this is the day she should start testing on (i.e. for a 26 day cycle, the estimated ovulation date would be day 13, subtract 3-4 days – so she should start testing on day 9 or 10 of her next menstrual cycle). A test should then be done every day until the rise in LH is picked up by the test.

These kits are widely available in chemists and some supermarkets and are simple to use. They consist of testing sticks, each day a different stick is placed in the urine stream. It is important that instructions for each kit are read carefully as timings vary with different kits. How the result is displayed can vary from different coloured lines through to smiley faces.

N.B. One word of caution here is that an LH surge does not guarantee ovulation. If there is an ovarian problem, the ovaries may not be able to respond to this surge.

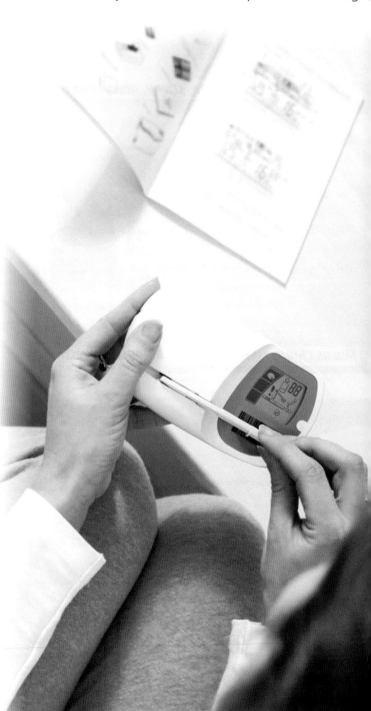

What can go wrong *with the natural process of fertility?*

Age

It is well known that as the female ages there is a decreased probability of conception and decreased ovarian reserve. However, the age of the male partner used to be considered to be less of an issue.

More recently, however, there have been studies that have shown that men's fertility decreases with age in the same way. According to one study of 782 couples, the level of sterility (no fertility present) stayed approximately the same in any of the age groups up to 40. But the 'time to pregnancy' rate in the other age groups (19-26, 27-29, 30-34, 35-39) all increased, indicating a lowering of fertility with increasing age.

Increased Infertility With Age in Men and Women David B. Dunson, Donna D. Baird, Bernardo Colombo, VOL. 103, NO. 1, JANUARY 2004 OBSTETRICS & GYNECOLOGY

This was the same in males and females. So there is a slow decline in fertility in both ages over time which of course starts to sharply drop in females as they are approaching the menopause. However, in men it does not have the same dramatic cut off point, so men can continue producing children into advanced age - it just might take them longer.

Effect of male age on fertility: evidence for the decline in male fertility with increasing age Mohamed A.M Hassan, Stephen R Killick, Fertility and Sterility Volume 79, Supplement 3, June 2003, Pages 1520–1527

Graph below reproduced from: NICE/National Collaborating Centre for Women's and Child Health. Fertility. NICE Clinical Guideline No. 156. London: NICE; 2013, with the permission of the Royal College of Obstetricians and Gynaecologists on behalf of NCC-WCH.

Calculated on the basis of studies in 10 different populations that did not use contraceptives (Heffner 2004[1], based on 2 reviews by Menken et al. 1986 and Anderson et al. 2000).

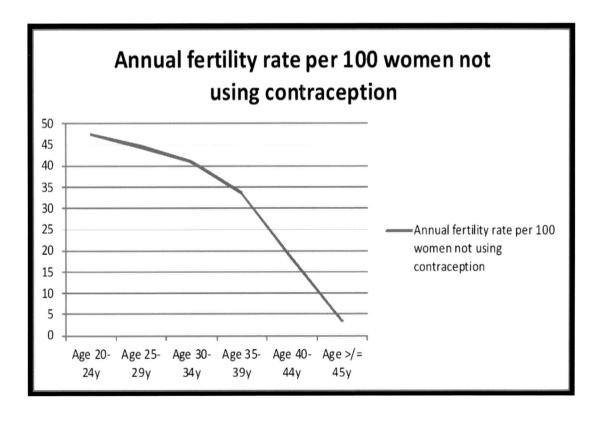

Main problems in fertility

Aside from the issues of age and stress, there are six main problems in fertility:

- blockages preventing the egg and sperm actually meeting.

- hormones at a less than optimal level.

- poor sperm or egg quality.

- absence of one or more parts of the reproductive system, or other physical issues.

- endometriosis / polycystic ovary syndrome.

- when conception can be natural but the baby carries a genetic problem.

Blockages preventing the egg and sperm from actually meeting

This is most commonly caused by blockages of connecting tubes in the reproductive organs - those of the fallopian tubes in the female and vas deferens tubes in the male. These tubes are lined with cilia, or finger-like projections which waft the egg or sperm in the right direction. If an infection occurs, the inflammation caused results in stickiness which can cause both sides of a tube to adhere so nothing can pass through the hole or lumen. This is particularly likely where there has been pelvic inflammatory disease in women. Occluded or blocked tubes can sometimes be cleared by use of surgery. There are also other causes of blockages such as tumours and variococeles (like varicose veins but on the scrotum) in men.

Sterilisation of women by 'tube tying or clipping' (tubal ligation) and vasectomy for men are classic examples of medically induced blockages. Sometimes these can be surgically reversed by cutting out the blocked areas and re-joining the tubes with some success, although IVF is quite often offered instead of surgery as it is so commonplace now. Female tubal ligation reversal has approximately a 50-60% success rate.

Vasectomy reversal rates are 55%, if it is reversed within 10 years, and approximately 25% after more than 10 years. There is no guarantee that fertility will return and there is usually a short window of opportunity for conception to take place – three to four months. If the two sex cells or gametes do not meet then pregnancy is not going to take place. Sometimes, there is an incomplete blockage which results in fertilisation

If the two sex cells or gametes do not meet then pregnancy is not going to take place. Sometimes, there is an incomplete blockage which results in fertilisation where the embryo gets stuck and embeds in the wrong

part of the organs; mainly this happens in the fallopian tube rather than the uterus. This causes an ectopic pregnancy which always results in the loss of the pregnancy and often the tube, which has to be removed by surgery as these pregnancies cannot possibly go to full term.

Usually, females with blocked tubes are offered IVF (see page 29), while males with blocked tubes are offered the PESA, MESA or TESA options (see page 33).

There can also be a problem with hostile cervical mucus. This blocks the sperm's entry to the cervix by having the wrong consistency, which in turn prevents the meeting of the egg and sperm. Treatment for this problem is usually IUI or IVF.

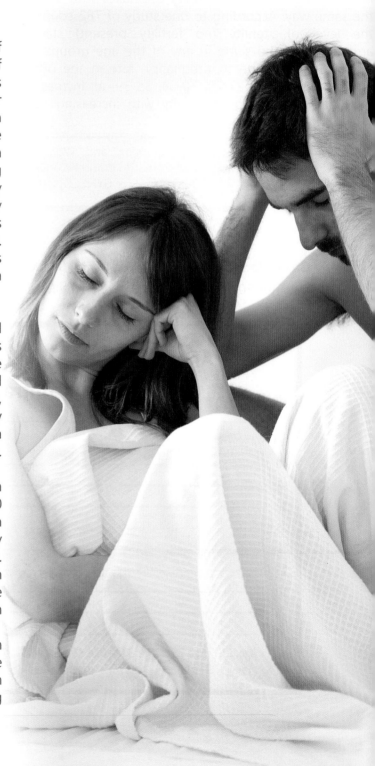

Hormones at less than optimum levels

Hormones are important in both the production of sperm and eggs. The female hormones are oestrogen, progesterone, follicle stimulating hormone (FSH) and Luteinising Hormone (LH). Men too have LH and FSH, but their main hormones are androgens. Androgens are steroid hormones, for example testosterone or dehydroepiandrosterone (DHEA), which control development and maintenance of masculine characteristics. There is also a reduced requirement for testosterone in females. Research on women with polycystic ovary syndrome (PCOS) suggests that high levels of androgens have a negative effect on female fertility as incidence of PCOS goes hand in hand with high testosterone and fertility problems. However, recent animal studies suggest correct amounts of FSH and androgens both need to occur and work together to bring about early follicle maturation.

The role of androgens in follicle maturation and ovulation induction: friend or foe of infertility treatment? Gleicher N, Weghofer A, Barad DH. Reproductive Biology and Endocrinology 2011;9(1):116

In the same way that testosterone is required in both males and females at different levels so is oestrogen. Oestrogen in women is very important as it is the primary female reproductive messenger and is central to the maturation of the follicle and egg production, while also helping to maintain bone formation and healthy cholesterol levels. Rising oestrogen levels in the menstrual cycle signals the production of FSH which in turn matures the egg. Increasing levels of oestrogen then triggers the release of Luteinising hormone (LH) which releases the mature egg. Oestrogen levels drop as progesterone levels peak. Progesterone performs better in the presence of oestrogen as the receptors for the progesterone molecules are upregulated when oestrogen is present.

Kastner P, Krust A, Turcotte B, Stropp U, Tora L, Gronemeyer H, Chambon P (1990). "Two distinct estrogen-regulated promoters generate transcripts encoding the two functionally different human progesterone receptor forms A and B". EMBO J. 9 (5): 1603–14.

Progesterone causes the uterine lining to thicken to become ready for the implantation of the embryo. During pregnancy, the placenta also produces high levels of progesterone after the first trimester. These levels drop at or shortly after birth, which may be involved in the onset of post natal depression (PND).

Hormonal predictors of postnatal depression at 6 months in breastfeeding women J. C. Ingram, R. J. Greenwood & M. W. Woolridge Journal of Reproductive and Infant Psychology Volume 21, Issue 1, 2003

Lack of oestrogen in males has h... be caused by disruption of...

Oestrogens in male reproc... Evan R. Simpson Best Pra... Endocrinology & Metabolism \... 505-516, September 2000

There are other hormones involv... to a lesser extent; however, the ... to have all the hormones working ... levels for communication with each oth...

Poor sperm

Egg Quality

The quality ... usually ava... This nearl... quality is ...

There a... or of ... hormo... three ... can i... prod... FSH ... Con... me... ca...

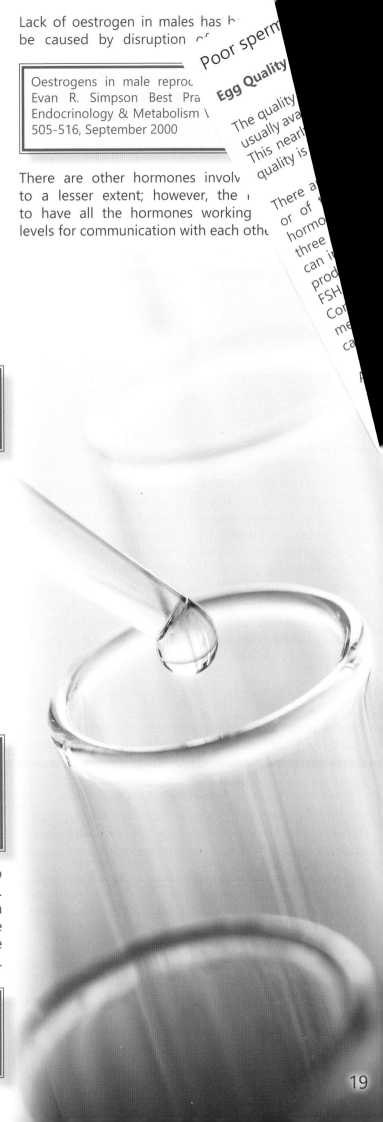

or egg quality

...of a woman's eggs is information that is not ...ilable until she has some form of egg retrieval. ...always happens after drug stimulation and ...mainly assessed by observation.

...re certain other indicators of poor egg quality ...the number of eggs available and these are ...nal. Follicle stimulating hormone (FSH) on day ...of the cycle is an indicator, a high level of FSH ...dicate poor eggs. This may be due to the ovary ...ucing less feedback (turn off) signals to the pituitary. ...controls the last two weeks of egg maturation. ...versely however, having a normal FSH does not ...an high quality eggs as high oestrogen levels ...n falsely reduce the concentration of the FSH.

Another test which is offered by some private clinics is the anti-Müllerian hormone concentration. anti-Müllerian hormone (AMH) is a hormone produced by the cells surrounding the egg in the follicle. These cells are called granulosa cells and the production of the hormone is at its strongest when the follicles are less than 4mm in size. AMH reduces as the follicle size increases and stops when the follicle reaches 8mm or more. This hormone production remains stable throughout the cycle so this test can be completed at any time in the cycle. A high production of this hormone can indicate polycystic ovary syndrome (PCOS). Medium production indicates good ovarian reserve - the presence of lots of small developing follicles. However, low levels tend to indicate poor ovarian reserve - few developing follicles present. AMH is an indicator of the early maturation process of the follicles.

http://www.advancedfertility.com/amh-fertility-test.htm

'From a research study it was shown that except at very young and very old ages, normal age specific-AMH better predicted higher oocyte yields than normal age specific-FSH, though above age 42 years normal age specific-FSH predicts good oocyte yields even with abnormally low AMH. Under age 42, discrepancies between age specific-FSH and age specific-AMH remain similarly predictive of oocyte yields at all ages.'

Discordances between follicle stimulating hormone (FSH) and anti-Müllerian hormone (AMH) in female infertility Norbert Gleicher, Andrea Weghofer, and David H Barad, Reprod Biol Endocrinol. 2010; 8: 64.

However, this test is not one that is offered by NHS hospitals as it is expensive, not completely proven and also has varying concentrations of AMH considered as 'normal' levels depending on the laboratory.

If your client has a diagnosis of poor ovarian reserve then they may become very upset; the idea of 'no eggs or poor eggs' is not attractive to women at any age, but when trying to become pregnant it can be destructive. Here, a listening ear can be very important. It is, however, fair to put a positive slant on this and point out that while they have reduced reserves they still have some reserves and where there are eggs, there are potential babies.

Where there are poor egg quality issues, the answer offered is often to use donor eggs.

One of the following measures will be used to predict the likely ovarian response to gonadotrophin stimulation in IVF:

- total antral follicle count of less than or equal to 4 for a low response and greater than 16 for a high response

- anti-Müllerian hormone of less than or equal to 5.4 pmol/l for a low response and greater than or equal to 25.0 pmol/l for a high response

- follicle-stimulating hormone greater than 8.9 IU/l for a low response and less than 4 IU/l for a high response.

National Institute for Health and Care Excellence (2013) Adapted from CG 156 Fertility: assessment and treatment for people with fertility problems. Manchester: NICE. Available from www.nice.org.uk/CG156 Reproduced with permission.

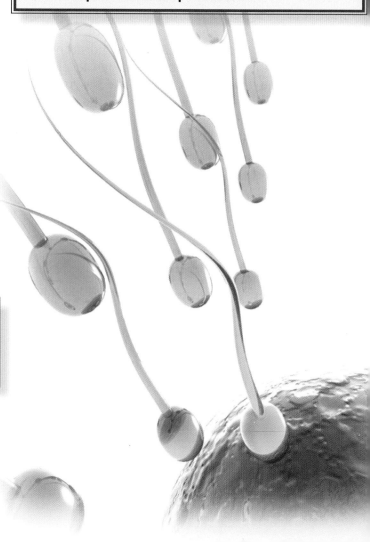

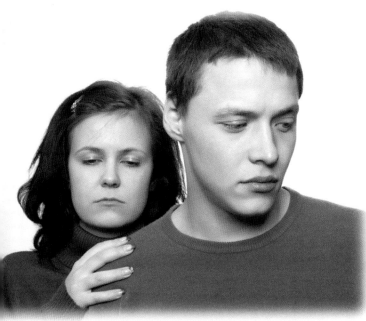

Sperm quality

Male factor issues are about 30% of all fertility problems. Depending on the problems with sperm quality/ quantity or motility (movement), there can be low levels (oligospermia), severely reduced levels (cryptoozospermia), or complete lack of sperm (azoospermia) in the ejaculate. These problems can all be easily detected by a simple sperm assessment. Normal sperm count is over 15 million per ml according to the World Health Organisation 2010, but older definitions state 20 million.

http://en.wikipedia.org/wiki/Semen_analysis

Table 1: Levels of low sperm count

Descriptor	Sperm concentrate in ejaculate
Mild Oligospermia	10 million to 20 million sperm/mL
Moderate Oligospermia	5 million to 10 million sperm/mL
Severe Oligospermia	0 to 5 million sperm/mL
Cryptoozospermia	0 - rare sperm
Azoospermia	0 sperm

http://theturekclinic.com/services/male-fertility/oligospermia/

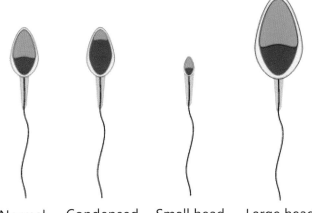

Normal   Condensed   Small head   Large head
              acrosome

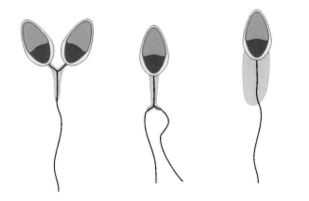

Double headed   Double tailed   Abnormal
                                  middle piece

There can also be morphological problems with the sperm. This means there are poorly formed or shaped sperm. A good sample would expect about 15% of all sperm to have normal morphology, but low morphology means that the choice of normal sperm is limited. Morphology problems can be two heads, bent tails or kinked mid sections. All of these cause problems with movement and with fertilisation.

If it is a poor sperm issue, the usual route of treatment would be to offer intra-cytoplasmic sperm injection or ICSI. If there are no sperm then the next route would be to look for blockages. If blockages are present then certain surgical procedures may be possible to retrieve sperm e.g. PESA, MESA and TESA. If, however, there is no production of viable sperm at all then donor sperm will be offered.

Picture by Xenzo at English Wikipedia

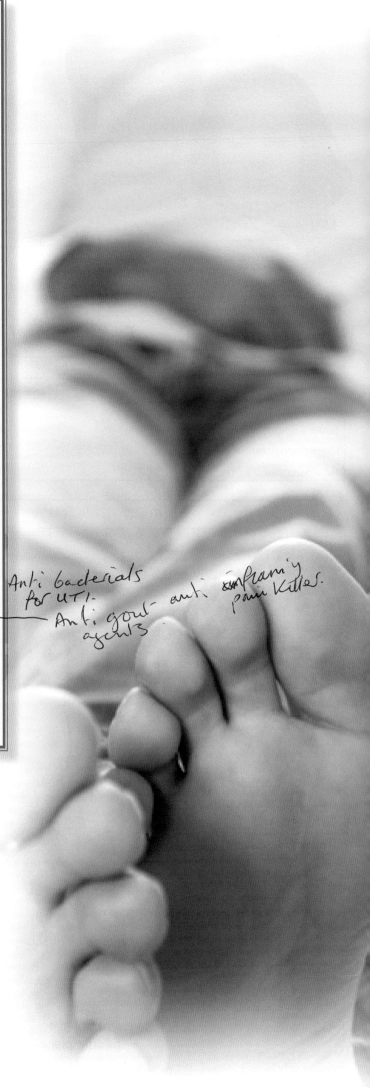

Advice from Patient UK on providing the ideal sample:

- Was the sample ideal? It may be worth repeating to check this. Was it taken to the laboratory in time? Was it kept warm? Cooling the sample or a delay in getting it to the laboratory can alter the number of active sperm and give a false result.

- High testes temperature. Sperm are made in the testes which are in the scrotum. This is the body's way of keeping the testes slightly cooler than the rest of the body, which is best for making sperm. It is often advised for men who have a low sperm count to wear loose-fitting underpants and trousers and to avoid very hot baths, saunas, etc. This aims to keep your testes slightly cooler than the rest of your body, which is thought to be good for sperm production. It is not clear whether these measures improve sperm count, but they seem to be sensible.

- Smoking can affect the sperm count. If you smoke, you should stop completely for optimum sperm production.

- Alcohol. More than 16 units per week (equivalent to about 8 pints of normal strength beer or 16 small glasses of wine) may interfere with optimum fertility.

- Drugs and medicines. Most do not interfere with sperm production, but some may do. These include: sulfasalazine, nitrofurantoin, tetracyclines, cimetidine, colchicine, allopurinol, some chemotherapy drugs, cannabis, cocaine and anabolic steroids. If you have a low sperm count, tell a doctor if you take any drugs or medicines regularly.

http://www.patient.co.uk/health/Semen-Analysis.htm

[handwritten annotations: Anti inflam chrones; Anti bacterials for UTI; Anti gout - anti inflam'y pain killer; Anti gout agents; Antiacid/Stomach H₂ blocker]

Remember: The whole process of sperm production takes 64 days and is very sensitive to changes in temperature, hormones and illness. The optimal temperature in men is two degrees below body temperature. Therefore, periods of raised temperature (for example a fever) can have a negative effect on sperm quality. So when a man has a poor sperm sample, it is worth thinking about what was happening 3 months before – was he ill or very stressed? This is why the diagnostic process usually requires more than one sample.

Absence of one or more component/physical issues

If one part of the reproductive system is missing or absent then it is probable that pregnancy will not take place. Complete absence of eggs, uterus or sperm would be an obvious problem and may result from medical interventions such as chemotherapy, surgery or from a birth defect. Exposure to radiation either medically or by accident can have a similar effect.

But there are other components that may be missing. For example, there is a condition called congenital bilateral absence of the vas deferens in males (CBAVD). This is a complete lack of the formation of the vas deferens (the tubes that transport the sperm from the testicles to the penis), bilateral meaning both sides. This condition often affects males carrying a defective gene involved in cystic fibrosis. For overt cystic fibrosis to be present, there needs to be a genetic mutation in both genes (i.e. both parents would have to carry the gene). With CBAVD, there is a mutation in only one gene and so not only can this be an indicator of a genetic carrier, but also possibly a previously unsuspected mild form of cystic fibrosis. Such men should be given tests to confirm or rule out such issues.

http://www.fertilityauthority.com/men-only/medical-causes-male-infertility/cbavd

In women, the most common cause of missing fallopian tubes is surgery, especially due to ectopic pregnancy.

The usual route around missing tubes is simply to go straight to IVF, whereas if the missing components are eggs or sperm, the customary answer is to go straight to donor. A missing uterus would require surrogacy.

There may also be problems with the process of reproduction, for example erectile dysfunction in men or vaginismus in women. Erectile dysfunction is where the process of erection is prevented in some way, for example due to a narrowing of the blood vessels (diabetes, high blood pressure, etc.), lack of hormones, or physical damage. Alternatively, psychological causes such as depression can have the same effect. Treatment can be provided by drugs for the underlying medical problem and also through using the circulation boosting drug Viagra. There are also vacuum pumps available to encourage blood flow. Cognitive behavioural therapy can be used when there are underlying psychological issues. If the routine treatments offered do not help this problem, then ICSI with surgical sperm collection may be used (PESA, MESA, TESA).

http://www.nhs.uk/conditions/Erectile-dysfunction/Pages/Introduction.aspx

Vaginismus is the involuntary clenching of the vaginal muscles when anything is inserted, making the physical side of reproduction very difficult and painful. Sometimes, this may arise from psychological issues caused by trauma. The most likely treatment for this would be by counselling or sex therapy.

http://www.nhs.uk/conditions/Vaginismus/Pages/Introduction.aspx

Self administration of sperm may overcome this problem without the need for IVF and it can be used in patients with this problem. But if IVF is required or preferred, certain stages of the IVF call for insertion of ultrasound guidance into the uterus. According to patient forums, it can help if the patient themselves does the placing of the probe as it allows for a level of control. The desire for a child can be strong enough to overcome the vaginismus hurdle. However, IVF may also bring past trauma to the fore which will need to be treated.

IVF in the Medically Complicated Patient: A Guide to Management By Nick S. Macklon

http://books.google.co.uk/books?id=HGM51_-hfE-IC&pg=PA74&lpg=PA74&dq=vaginismus+IVF&source=bl&ots=8gPUuB7cY2&sig=IKaBzRKkbXfxVuQh-pSk8HCBMa1I&hl=en&sa=X&ei=L9P3ULDSA82ChQeKz-oCYBw&ved=0CE0Q6AEwAg#v=onepage&q=vaginismus%20IVF&f=false

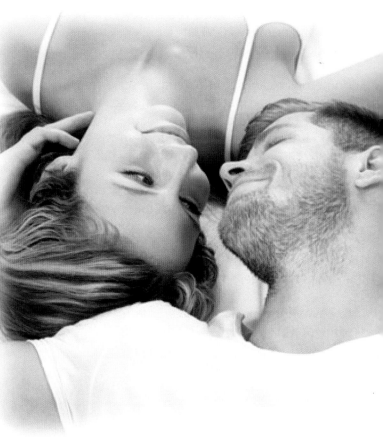

Endometriosis/ Polycystic ovary syndrome (PCOS)

Endometriosis

This is where cells of the endometrial lining become embedded in other areas of the abdominal cavity, most commonly around the pelvis; these are called endometrial implants. These cells continue to undergo the same changes under the action of hormones as they would if they were still in the uterine cavity. The tissues break down and eventually bleed when progesterone levels drop, which causes inflammation because there is nowhere for the shed endometrial tissue to go. This inflammation can cause scarring and stickiness, or adhesions to form which - depending on where the implants are - can cause areas full of naturally moving organs to become attached to one another and therefore immobile. Endometrial tissue can also form cysts on the ovary (called chocolate cysts due to the way they look). All together, these issues usually result in extreme pain, fatigue, depression and difficulty with sex. There is an increased rate of infertile women with endometriosis but it is unclear whether the underlying problems with the endometrium being elsewhere causes infertility or if the underlying problems with fertility cause the endometrium to wander.

http://books.google.co.uk/books?id=HGM51_-hfE IC&pg=PA74&lpg=PA74&dq=vaginismus+IVF& source=bl&ots=8gPUuB7cY2&sig=IKaBzRKkbXfx VuQhpSk8HCBMa1I&hl=en&sa=X&ei=L9P3ULD SA82ChQeKzoCYBw&ved=0CE0Q6AEwAg#v=onep age&q=vaginismus%20IVF&f=false
(see page 103).

Endometriosis can be on a variable scale from mild to severe. Where the patient is on this scale will decide what sort of standard medical treatment they will be offered. If there is only mild endometriosis then it may be managed symptomatically with pain relief, hormone treatments or going on the pill. For more advanced stages, there are surgical treatments from key hole surgery (laparoscopy) up a to full hysterectomy in very severe cases. In the former a laser or other heat source is used to destroy the endometrial implants. The decision of treatment course will take into account the woman's age, symptoms and fertility needs.

http://www.nhs.uk/Conditions/Endometriosis/Pages/Treatment.aspx

Endometriosis is the third most likely cause for the requirement of assisted conception. Where there are adhesions present in the abdominal cavity, there can be problems with fallopian tube movement and the natural egg transfer to the fallopian tubes. Controlled ovarian stimulation with intrauterine sperm injection (COS-IUI) has been used but for severe cases of endometriosis the likely treatment offered will be IVF.

Polycystic ovary syndrome (PCOS)

This is one of the main causes of female subfertility, resulting in 5-10% of all infertility cases. It is potentially genetically linked as a PCOS patient is more likely to have a female relation with the same problem. PCOS is a syndrome which means that an individual with PCOS may exhibit any number of a list of symptoms, from two or three to the entire list. They do, however, diagnostically have to have cysts present on the ovaries. Cysts form when something has gone wrong hormonally with the maturation of the ovarian follicles, so the eggs do not mature and are not released.

Symptoms:

- Presence of ovarian cysts
- Reduced number of periods each year
- Fertility problems
- Weight gain
- Hirsutism: excess hair in places not expected in a female
- Thinning of hair on the scalp: male baldness pattern
- Acne
- Problems with blood sugar
- Depression

These symptoms are caused by:

- Insulin resistance – problems with the sensitivity of cells to insulin, which in turn can cause high levels of insulin
- Hormonal imbalances; especially high Luteinising hormone and testosterone levels and low levels of sex binding globulin.
- Weight gain could possibly be due to the high circulating blood sugar levels, resulting from insulin resistance, which will then be converted to body fat
- Genetics; having female relations with PCOS increases the probability.

Treatment of PCOS is symptomatic. Weight loss of even 5% can lead to a lessening of symptoms. A medication called Metformin commonly used in the treatment of diabetes is used to help the insulin resistance. Cream can be used to reduce hair growth. Surgery can be used to reduce the number of cysts - ovarian drilling or diathermy may be provided when the other treatments have not worked. Hormone treatment in the form of the pill can be used but of course this doesn't help if pregnancy is desired.

http://www.verity-pcos.org.uk/guide_to_pcos/what_is_pcos.

http://www.patient.co.uk/health/Polycystic-Ovary-Syndrome.htm

http://www.nhs.uk/Conditions/Polycystic-ovarian-syndrome/Pages/Treatment.aspx

For a woman with PCOS who is trying to get pregnant, the most likely route to be offered will be IVF. It might seem that someone with lots of follicles on their ovaries would have lots of eggs under stimulation but the outcome of IVF with PCOS is comparable to any other IVF patient.

http://humrep.oxfordjournals.org/content/14/1/167.full

When conception may be capable of occurring naturally but embryos are being specifically chosen

Genetically carried illnesses – this is a rare scenario but you need to be aware of it.

When there is potential for a genetic problem to be carried through the gametes to cause a serious medical illness as a newborn, in childhood or even as an adult, unaffected embryos may be chosen using IVF and pre implantation genetic diagnosis. Typical examples of diseases are Spinal Muscular Atrophy (SMA) which affects babies, Duchenne Muscular Dystrophy (DMD) which affects young children through to teenagers and Huntingdon's disease (HD) which is late adult onset, all of which are passed through generations via a mutation in a gene. Often, it is not known that a family has an inherited disease until at least one child has been born with it; however, with the adult onset inherited diseases there are situations where the affected adult may already have grown up children before the disease is diagnosed This then becomes an issue for the next generation. In most cases of genetic disease, provided the mutation causing the disease has been discovered and is testable in the family line, it is possible to offer pre-implantation

genetic diagnosis. This is where a single cell from an embryo grown in vitro can be removed by careful manipulation, leaving the remainder of the embryo intact and continuing to grow. These single cells can then be investigated using a complicated process of multiplying the DNA and then searching for the disease causing mutation. Where the mutation is not present, the embryo can be transferred to the mother to be carried in the normal way, which hopefully results in a healthy baby. Sometimes, for example in the Y-chromosome inherited diseases, it can be as simple as only putting back females as the illness would only be present in the males.

This method of treatment does, however, turn reproduction which might happen naturally into an unnatural and very costly process. In these cases there is an even greater likelihood of emotional involvement. There may also be the added stresses of unwell children or other family members.

http://www.hfea.gov.uk/preimplantation-genetic-diagnosis.html

Saviour siblings

These are babies that are specifically selected at embryo level to match the tissue type of an unwell sibling. The stem cells that are retrievable from the baby's cord blood can be used to provide a transplant for children with inheritable illnesses or other spontaneous illnesses such as Beta thallassaemia and Diamond Blackfan anaemia. The embryos are tested using the same pre-implantation diagnostic techniques and then tissue typed to find a match for the sibling. As you can imagine, this situation comes with many levels of fear and worry.

http://www.hfea.gov.uk/preimplantation-tissue-typing.html

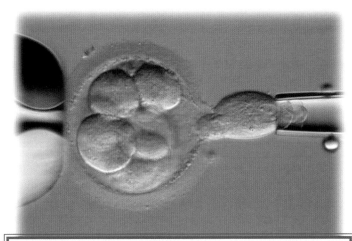

Embryo being biopsied at 8 cell stage, courtesy of Dr P Renwick, Centre for Preimplantation Genetic Diagnosis, Guy's Hospital, London UK

Defining tests: *what your clients have been going through*

First of all, it is important to be aware of where your clients are in their fertility journey. They might just be starting out with a vague idea that it's taking longer than they expected - or, at the other end of the scale, they might have tried everything and you are their last hope. Whatever the situation, it is important to manage your client's expectations; you are supporting them through this journey, not treating the fertility problem - and anything else will be a bonus!

If they are at the beginning of the journey, then you need to keep in mind how long they have been trying and the age of the female in the equation.

> People who are concerned about their fertility should be informed that over 80% of couples in the general population will conceive within 1 year if: the woman is aged under 40 years and they do not use contraception and have regular sexual intercourse. Of those who do not conceive in the first year, about half will do so in the second year (cumulative pregnancy rate over 90%).
>
> A woman of reproductive age who has not conceived after 1 year of unprotected vaginal sexual intercourse, in the absence of any known cause of infertility, should be offered further clinical assessment and investigation along with her partner. Offer an earlier referral for specialist consultation to discuss the options for attempting conception, further assessment and appropriate treatment where: the woman is aged 36 years or over there is a known clinical cause of infertility or a history of predisposing factors for infertility.
>
> **National Institute for Health and Care Excellence (2013) Adapted from CG 156 Fertility: assessment and treatment for people with fertility problems. Manchester: NICE. Available from www.nice.org.uk/CG156 Reproduced with permission.**

If your couple has been trying for a while – and this means really trying, not like the couples who live international lifestyles and spend part of the month apart for business reasons and just happen to miss the fertile window every month - then it is worth urging them to go to their doctor to have tests just to rule out any problems. No matter how great you are at reflexology, you will never be able to help a couple that have blocked fallopian tubes and no sperm!

It is also worth sensitively checking that the woman knows when she is most likely to be fertile; are they

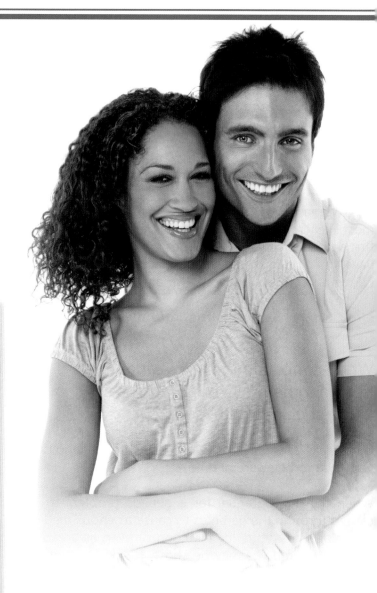

aware of the fertile window? If they don't know when they are fertile, they could be missing it every month and sometimes just getting them together at the right time can make a difference.

If they are the international traveller type of couple, then it is also worth just checking how many times in the period they have been trying that they were actually in the same place for the fertile period. It can be enlightening for them to find out that although they think they have been trying for 8 months, they have actually only been in the same place at the right time for 3 of those months. It can help calm a lot of fears.

There is also sometimes a bit of a lag immediately after stopping taking the pill before the female regains fertility, possibly taking a few months to regain her natural rhythm and again this should be factored in.

If the couple have been trying properly for a while, then recommend they visit their GP. Here they will be given both male and female tests to define if there is anything wrong on a biological level. After a range of tests, about 25% of all couples will be given a diagnosis of idiopathic or unexplained fertility; they may be offered treatment or not, or may decline further treatment - but at least they will know the situation.

Blood tests

This is the first line of testing and the blood is taken on specific days of the cycle. If the female's cycle is irregular, the blood needs to be taken around the right days. The tests are usually on day 3 and day 21 or about 7 days before the expected date of the period. The blood taken will be tested for oestrogen, progesterone, follicle stimulating hormone (FSH) and luteinising hormone (LH). This will give a decent hormone profile picture. Other hormones like testosterone and prolactin may also be measured.

There is one other hormone test which is sometimes carried out by the private clinics - the anti-Müllerian hormone test (AMH test). This checks for the production of the hormone that comes from small immature follicles and can be an indicator of ovarian reserve – or how many eggs are left.

Chlamydia will probably also be tested for, either by a urine based test or by a swab. It is important to know whether Chlamydia is present because it can not only indicate possible pelvic inflammatory disease, but can also cause problems with the IVF process. Treatment is easy with antibiotics.

http://www.hfea.gov.uk/fertility-basics.html

Thyroid testing

Thyroid problems have been shown to be related to miscarriage so often tests are carried out to check for thyroid efficiency. Treatment would be as normal for a thyroid problem.

Anti-phospholipid antibodies

Antibodies to molecules that are usually found on cells, called phospholipids are sometimes found in patients with Lupus or Rheumatoid Arthritis and if the antibodies are known to be present they can be monitored and treated. Sometimes they are found in people without these diseases and they are diagnosed as having antiphospholipid (or Hughes) syndrome, or as having 'too sticky blood'. These antibodies can cause the blood to clot too fast and this can result in many problems including problems with implantation and the development of the placenta in pregnancy. Often treatment is simply a low dose of Aspirin but may also have to involve other anti-coagulants or other medicine.

http://www.hughes-syndrome.org/about-hughes-syndrome/hughes.php

Reproductive immunology

This is the science of the immune system and how the implantation of an embryo which is partially foreign (the father's DNA) is permissible. The immune system usually protects the body from invasion by foreign bodies, viruses, bacteria and foreign tissue. It naturally repels anything it sees as not self. However in the case of pregnancy this is allowed to happen due to active toleration of the foreign element carried on the placenta forming cells, by the immune system. Natural killer cells are present in everyone all of the time and have a specific role in combatting infections, a decrease in natural killer (NK) cells is thought to play a large part in the implantation process. When the levels of NK cells raise so the risk of pregnancy failure increases. Tests can be carried out to check the levels of NK activity in women with recurrent miscarriages.

The new treatment for this problem is a mixture of steroids – to reduce the cytotoxic effects of the cells and intra-lipid (large fat molecule) infusions usually every two weeks. These are a mixture of egg yolk, soya oil, glycerine and water which is given by intra-venous infusion directly into the circulation and is thought to strengthen the cell membranes to protect against NK cell action or to modulate the NK cell action, although how intra-lipid works is not really understood. Small studies have shown that this treatment can radically increase the probability of pregnancy.

Normally large fat molecules like egg yolk are passed into the body via breakdown in the digestive system but in this situation they are being infused into the circulation and this is not a normal process. It is not known how reflexology will affect this but if we think about what reflexology aims to do – to remove waste products – then there could be a tendency for the body to move the large molecules to the liver for breakdown more readily. But to do their job the large lipid molecules need to remain in the circulation so reflexology might be acting against what is best for the client. Because this whole area of treatment is very new, for now we would recommend that reflexology is not provided whilst intra-lipid infusion treatment is ongoing.

Does Immunotherapy for Treatment of Reproductive Failure Enhance Live Births? Carolyn B. Coulam1 , Brian Acacio American Journal of Reproductive Immunology 67 (2012) 296-303

Tube tests

The next test that will be done is to check for working fallopian tubes.

Hysteriosalpingogram. This is where a dye is inserted through the vagina and into the uterus. It is high contrast dye, which means it can be viewed under X-ray to check that the dye passes up through the uterus and out through the fallopian tubes.

Hystero Contrast Sonography (HyCoSy) is an ultrasound procedure intended to diagnose structural defects of the female reproductive system, such as blockage of the fallopian tubes. It is conducted by forcing an aqueous fluid up the fallopian tube to provide a contrast medium for ultrasound.

Both of these tests check that the egg can pass in the opposite direction and that there are no blockages. Any further problems discovered will then need to be investigated by laparoscopy (key hole surgery) of the abdominal cavity.

Sperm tests

The male will be asked to provide a sperm sample; this usually happens in the clinic, although if this causes problems it can be provided at home and transported into the clinic - but it needs to arrive in less than one hour and to have been kept at body temperature, as time and temperature will affect the viability of the sample. If getting the sample in the pot provided causes problems, there is the possibility of using a condom, but these have to be specially provided by the fertility clinic as they must not include spermicide.

Post coital test

This is a test that is often carried out when there is no problem with the sperm concentration, or with the hormones, tube, patency or ovulation in the female. There is the possibility that there is an immune problem between the couple. The cervical mucus in the female changes around ovulation and becomes thinner and more like egg white, allowing passage of the sperm through the cervix; however, occasionally this can become thick at the wrong time and prevent the passage of the sperm though the cervix. There is also a possibility where the mucus gains antibodies to the male partner's sperm. The antibodies can cause the sperm to clump together, which prevents them from penetrating the mucus and reaching the egg. So even though the sperm sample is acceptable, on meeting the mucus it becomes non-viable.

This test involves the collection of cervical mucus by an examination 2-8 hours after intercourse around the time of ovulation. The mucus is observed under a microscope to check for the viability of the sperm present.

http://www.ncbi.nlm.nih.gov/pubmed/68329

http://www.fertilitycommunity.com/fertility/post-coital-test-for-infertility-diagnosis.html

There is also the chance that the male has produced antibodies against his own sperm. This occasionally happens after injury or surgery to the testicles and is where the body reacts against itself (auto-immune reaction). These antibodies can result in dead or deformed sperm.

http://www.medicalhealthtests.com/antibody-tests/antisperm-antibodies-test.html

If any of these problems are detected, steroids may be prescribed to reduce antibody concentration, but it is more likely that the answer will be to go straight to IVF.

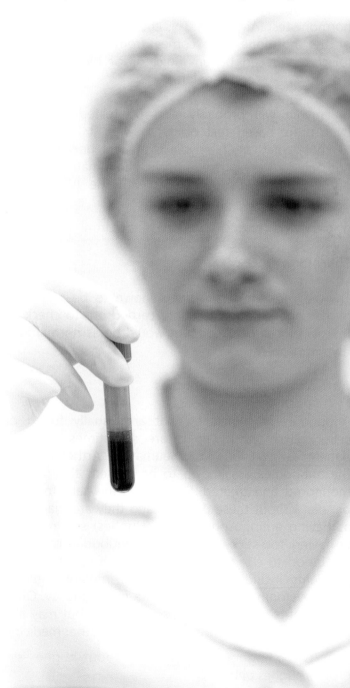

Assisted conception techniques

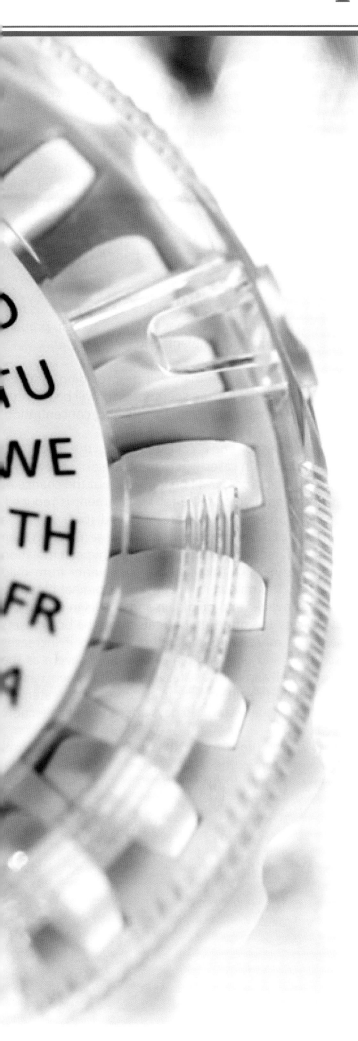

Assisted conception treatments for infertility are actually quite few:

- Drug stimulation with natural conception

- Drug stimulation with assisted conception

- Soft IVF or Natural cycle assisted conception

Usually the first two are used in order; the final one is only used in some more specialised clinics.

Within the assisted conception arena, there are several possible routes depending on where the fertility issue lies - female, male or both.

Drug stimulation with natural cycle conception

Clomid

If there is an issue with ovulation in the female and no problems with the male, this is usually the first port of call. An uncomplicated female under 40 would be prescribed Clomid or Clomiphene citrate which is a straightforward ovulation inducing drug to make the brain produce more FSH. It is given in tablet form for the first five days of the cycle. It is a competitive inhibitor of oestrogen. It stimulates the pituitary gland to produce follicle stimulating hormone (FSH), which in turn will stimulate the ovaries to mature a follicle or multiple follicles containing eggs. Oestrogen normally has a negative effect on the pituitary: Clomid blocks oestrogen and leads to pituitary FSH production and ovarian stimulation. During treatment it is of course necessary for regular intercourse to take place. This allows for natural cycle conception, although sometimes it might be that the best route is to have intrauterine insemination (IUI) as well.

http://theadventurouswriter.com/blogbaby/what-is-clomid-how-does-clomid-help-you-get-pregnant/

Intrauterine sperm injection (IUI)

This is used when there is a potential problem that the sperm is not getting to the right place at the right time. It is often used when there are problems with sperm movement (motility), sperm concentration, hostile mucus at the cervix or problems with maintenance of an erection. The sperm is collected and concentrated and then placed in the uterus at the right time in the natural cycle or during a stimulated cycle if it is necessary. Either way, the release of the egg will be monitored using ultrasound and the sperm inserted 36-40 hours after ovulation. Unlike with IVF, the egg is not removed from the uterus in this process; it stays in situ.

This same process can also be used with donor sperm.

Drug stimulation with assisted conception

This falls into several categories but all entail some sort of drug stimulation followed by removal and manipulation of the eggs and/or sperm.

In Vitro Fertilisation (IVF)

In vitro literally translates from latin as 'in glass' and while it is usually thought of as being carried out in a test tube, actually the technique is performed with each egg in a separate bubble of sterile fluid located under a clear oil in a flat dish, called a Petri dish.

IVF is usually required when there is impaired female function but adequate sperm function.

Downregulation

The process usually starts with the female having her own cycle suppressed by taking drugs such as Burserelin and Goserelin, which copy the action of natural hormones that block the release of the two hormones controlling ovulation: FSH and LH. These are known as gonadotrophin releasing hormone (GnRH) analogues. These are taken as a nasal spray or as a daily or monthly injection before, or at the same time as, fertility drugs. During this time she may feel like she is going through menopausal symptoms, which is actually what is happening, only the hormones are being artificially decreased rather than naturally decreased by the body.

Stimulation

Once the natural cycle is low enough, the reproductive system can then be artificially stimulated to kick start the ovaries back to action. Drugs containing follicle stimulating hormone (FSH) and/or luteinising hormone (LH) stimulate the ovaries to produce mature eggs. These include Gonal-f, Puregon, Menogon, Menopur and Merional. They are injected into a muscle or under the skin by clinic staff. However, injection at home is usually possible. When the eggs are ready, a single injection of the hormone human Chorionic Gonadotrophin (hCG), called a priming injection, is given to mature the eggs.

Egg collection

At this point the woman is brought into the clinic and given either sedation or general anaesthetic. A large needle is then passed up the vagina and through the wall of the uterus under ultrasound guidance into the maturing follicles. Mature eggs are collected or 'harvested' and transferred into a test tube of fluid containing medium (artificial compounds mimicking human fluids). Each egg is then transferred under a microscope into its own individual drop of medium under a film of oil and placed in an incubator at body temperature.

On the day of egg collection the woman will usually be given uterine progesterone pessaries to help prepare the endometrium for implantation.

At the same time, the male will be providing a sperm sample. As for the IUI, the sperm present will be counted and then washed and diluted to a suitable concentration.

If there are no eggs collected then the cycle will be abandoned. In cases where there are only a few eggs collected, the process will be followed but the chance of having an embryo suitable for replacement is reduced. If large numbers of eggs are retrieved (over 20), or a high level of oestrogen results from the stimulation then there is a higher chance of ovarian hyperstimulation syndrome (OHSS). This can vary in severity from mild to severe. The mild version causes abdominal bloating, enlarged ovaries and mild pain and occurs in about 1 in 3 IVF cycles. It is often left untreated and the body resets itself. The more serious situation is when it increases in severity and danger. Pain can become severe as the ovaries swell and fluid (ascites) fills the abdomen; nausea and vomiting result and it can become life threatening. Symptoms usually start 4-5 days after the egg collection.

http://www.patient.co.uk/doctor/Ovarian-Hyperstimulation-Syndrome.htm

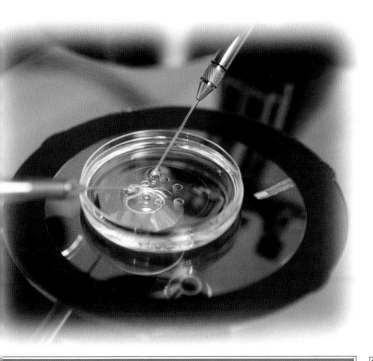

Introduction of sperm into bubble of fluid (medium) containing a single egg.

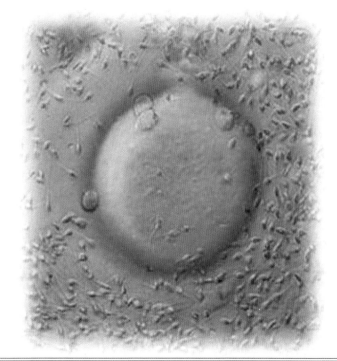

Picture courtesy of Dr P Renwick, Centre for Preimplantation Genetic Diagnosis, Guy's Hospital, London UK

In vitro fertilisation technique

A certain number of sperm will be introduced to each fluid bubble containing an egg. These are then left to themselves overnight.

During the maturation process, the egg contains two sets of chromosomes, containing two 'X' sex chromosomes. During egg maturation the second unwanted set of chromosomes is extruded into a polar body and becomes inactive leaving one set of chromosomes in the egg. The sperm then provides the second set of chromosomes during fertilisation which has either an X or Y sex chromosome to provide a female or male baby – XX female, XY male.

The egg and a single sperm interact and fertilisation takes place.

Day 1 the cells will have joined and then cleaved (split into two cells). This is the beginning of new life. It is also the most likely point where the embryos can 'arrest' or stop growing.

Day 2 the two cells split into four and then again into eight

Day 3 the eight cells split again into 16 and then into 32 - at this point the developing organism is called a morula.

Day 4 the morula compacts into a ball of cells so that each individual cell cannot be distinguished.

Day 5 - 6 the cells separate into two different cell layers with a visible cavity; the layer on the inside is going to be the baby and and the one on the outside will be the placenta. This is called a blastocyst.

At any point the embryos can arrest (stop growing). This is usually because there have been chromosome mistakes in the embryos, making them non-viable.

Embryo transfer

Transfer of the embryo back into the female is usually carried out at the eight cell stage or the blastocyst stage. Which stage embryo transfer occurs in is linked to how many embryos are available; the more available, the more likely that even if some stop growing on days 4 and 5 there will still be some that reach blastocyst stage. Implantation is more likely to happen if the embryo is returned at the blastocyst stage simply because it is further through the developmental process. Transfer is achieved by sucking up the embryo under the microscope into a thin tube or catheter and passing it through the vagina, into the uterus where the embryo is then released.

Hatching and Implantation

At this point the embryo floats free in the uterus. The zona pellucida around the egg now becomes constraining rather than protective, so enzymes start to break down the protein, allowing the embryo to squeeze its way out. Next, the cells on the surface of the blastocyst change, becoming enlarged and sticky (trophoblast cells). The endometrium is also undergoing changes, producing decidual cells and pinopodes – these cells reduce the volume of fluid in the uterus, allowing the embryo to be closer to the walls and therefore more likely to stick. The trophoblast cells change to giant cells which then escape from the embryo and start to invade into the surface of the endometrium, resulting in attachment and eventually the setting up of a circulatory system that becomes the placenta. During the establishment of the pregnancy, it is possible that there may be slight breakthrough bleeding.

31

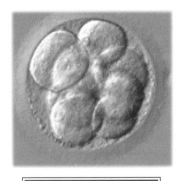

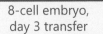
8-cell embryo,
day 3 transfer

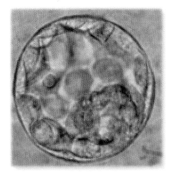
blastocyst,
day 5 transfer

Human Chorionic Gonadotrophin (hCG) is produced by the invading cells from the embryo - this is what is measured in a pregnancy test and is what defines pregnancy. There is a required time frame from fertilisation to implantation to allow sufficient build-up of HCG for the body to recognise it is pregnant. This occurs about 14 days after egg collection or ovulation in non assisted cycles.

If implantation doesn't succeed, the pregnancy test will be negative. Progesterone levels drop, the endometrium sloughs off and the woman has a period. If it succeeds and a positive pregnancy test happens, the next stage to get to is the 6 weeks scan which (amongst other things) checks for the presence of a heartbeat. This indicates a viable pregnancy but and also shows if there are multiple pregnancies present.

After a positive cardiac scan, the next milestone is the standard 12 week scan and this is where the IVF pregnancy is then transferred over to normal antenatal care.

Prevention of multiple births

In women up to the age of 40 a maximum of 2 embryos are transferred; after 40, three may be transferred if there is a good reason to do so. However, there is a policy in the UK for offering elective single embryo transfer or e-SET. If there are very high quality embryos available and there are no concerns over other aspects of the pregnancy, single embryo transfer may be offered. This does not necessarily mean that only a single baby will result as there is a very tiny percentage of embryos that will spilt to become monozygotic or identical twins, but it does hugely reduce the chance of multiple births, which is better for the health of both the mother and resulting babies.

http://www.hfea.gov.uk/2587.html#3050

All images on this page courtesy of Dr P Renwick, Centre for Preimplantation Genetic Diagnosis, Guy's Hospital, London UK

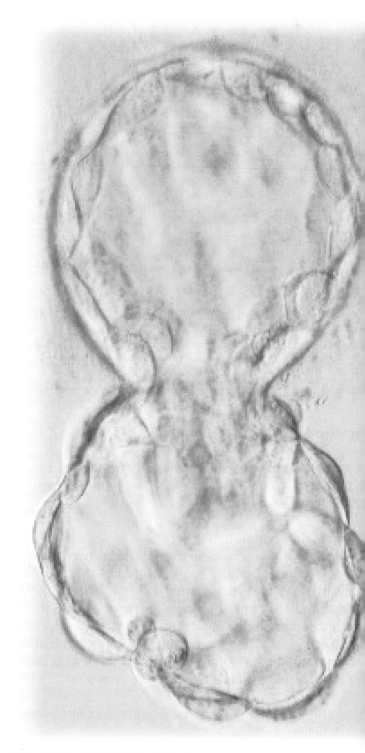

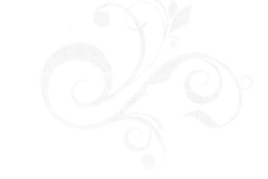
Hatching embryo; upper part includes the zona pellucida

Intra cytoplasmic sperm injection (ICSI)

This is used when there are male factor problems, usually when there are low levels of normal sperm in the ejaculate. The female undergoes the standard IVF procedure while the man produces a sample. The difference is that that once the eggs are collected, the sperm is put into a dish and individual normal or healthy looking sperm are selected into an extremely thin glass tube. Each egg is very carefully held against a tube using suction to keep it in place, while an individual sperm is gently injected into the middle of the nucleus of the egg. After this, the egg is returned back into its drop of medium under the oil and the same process as for standard IVF is followed. Where there are issues of difficulties with ejaculation, it is possible to have the sample provided earlier and frozen to prevent the possibility of the female undergoing egg collection with no sperm available for fertilisation. http://www.hfea.gov.uk/ICSI.html

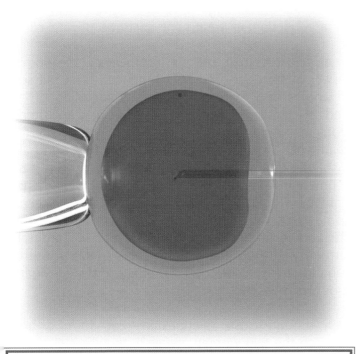

Sperm injection to a single egg using the ICSI technique

Pre-implantation genetic diagnosis (PGD)

Where there are genetically transmitted illnesses in a family, for example spinal muscular atrophy (SMA) or Huntingdon's disease (HD) it is possible to have a further stage inserted into the IVF procedure where one cell is removed from the 8 cell embryo and tested specifically for the familial genetic mutation (where there is a specific change in the DNA that results in the disease). All the cells in the embryo prior to separation into the two blastocyst layers are totipotent (they have the ability to become any cell in the body), therefore removing one at this stage does not seem to affect the embryo in any way. The embryo is held and a fine tube is inserted;

one cell is sucked out and placed into a small tube, while the embryo is returned back to its droplet under oil and left to recover and keep dividing. The one cell and its single strand of DNA is then put through a series of steps where the DNA is multiplied to provide millions of copies of the individual DNA strand, which are then tested for the specific mutation of that disease as found in their family. The embryos free from the mutation will then be grown on and the best one or two will be returned. This is the same process as is used for saviour sibling selection.

http://www.hfea.gov.uk/preimplantation-genetic-diagnosis.html

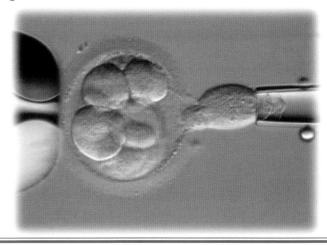

Single cell removal from an eight cells embryo for pre-implantation genetic diagnosis, courtesy of Dr P Renwick, Centre for Preimplantation Genetic Diagnosis, Guy's Hospital, London UK

Situations of no sperm or very low sperm in the ejaculate

This may be the case if there are problems with the production of sperm or more likely blockages or absences of tubes. In these cases the sperm is collected from different parts of the male reproductive system by using different techniques and then, because of the low levels of sperm collected, is usually used in ICSI.

These surgical collection techniques are called MESA, PESA, TESA and for the more extreme situations TESE:

- PESA: percutaneous epididymal sperm aspiration.
- MESA: microsurgical epididymal sperm aspiration.
- TESA: testicular sperm aspiration
- TESE: testicular sperm extraction. This involves opening up the scrotum and taking a large volume of testicular tissue, perhaps from several regions of the testicle. Sperm are then retrieved using a microscope to identify individual sperm.

Many of the sperm retrieved by these techniques are immature and so cannot be used for standard IVF – instead they have to be used in the ICSI process.

http://fertility.treatmentabroad.com/treatments/surgical-sperm-retrieval-pesa-tesa-mesa

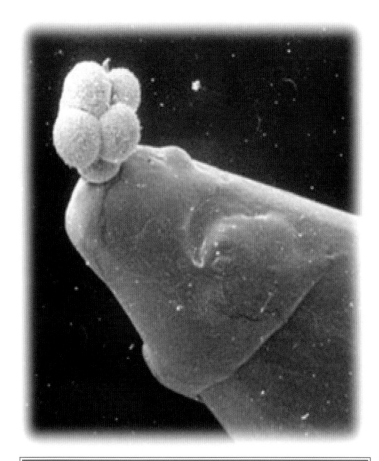

Embryo on a pin head without the zona pellucida
courtesy of George Nikos

Freezing of gametes and embryos

Sometimes there is a need for the gametes (the sperm and eggs) to be frozen. Sperm has been successfully frozen for many years; however, the freezing of eggs is still a relatively new technique.

The freezing of eggs usually only takes place where there is a medical treatment approaching which will destroy female fertility – this is usually related to cancer treatment. The freezing of eggs has only been carried out for the last ten years and the thawing of eggs is not very successful.

http://www.hfea.gov.uk/46.html

There is also the choice of freezing ovarian tissue but this is also a relatively new technique.

Either way, the freezing takes place in liquid nitrogen and storage is time limited to about 10 years. The frozen gametes (egg and sperm) legally belong to the individual.

When it comes to the freezing of embryos, this is much more successful than the freezing of eggs, and often if there are good remaining embryos left after transfer then the freezing option will be offered. Some embryos will not survive the thawing process, so it is only worth freezing them if there are a few available. These can be replaced into a natural cycle or a prepared cycle as

obviously there is no need for the full IVF stimulation during a frozen embryo transfer cycle. There is no evidence that the frozen embryos are less likely to be viable or result in a pregnancy than fresh embryo transfers.

Legally, the frozen embryos belong to the couple as they each have a 50% DNA input. This is OK until a marriage or partnership breaks down; if this happens, the embryos must not be used without consent of the other partner.

http://humrep.oxfordjournals.org/content/15/5/979.full

Donor eggs, sperm and surrogacy

Where there is a situation of poor egg or sperm quality to the extent that it is unlikely that pregnancy will result, the route of choice may be donor gametes. In the UK it is illegal to pay for donations of either and so the availability of each is purely due to altruism. It is possible to choose certain genetic characteristics that match the couple involved, for example hair, skin and eye colour. Sometimes donor eggs have been given in exchange for a reduction in treatment costs at private clinics.

When it comes to a uterine insufficiency, the obvious answer is surrogacy; however, this can bring all sorts of worries and fears to the fore. Depending on the medical problems present, a woman with uterine problems may still be able to undergo fertility treatment, which would allow her eggs and her husband's sperm to produce the embryos even if she is not able to physically carry the pregnancy. These embryos would then be transferred into a second woman's uterus for the term of the pregnancy. This situation is termed gestational surrogacy. Traditional surrogacy is where the male partners sperm is inserted using IUI into the surrogate's uterus and the surrogate's eggs are fertilised.

Even though close relationships can form a bond between the two women involved, there is still often a fear that the baby will not handed over at birth. The law in the UK states that a fee and expenses can be paid and it is a good idea to have an agreed contract signed in advance.

http://humupd.oxfordjournals.org/content/9/5/483.full.pdf

Soft IVF/ Natural cycle conception

These techniques are becoming favoured in women that are nearing the end of their fertile state, when the body does not react well to high concentrations of drugs.

Soft IVF uses low levels of stimulatory drugs on a natural cycle, so the woman's own cycle is not downregulated or suppressed. This reduces the concentration of drugs required and reduces the cost, while minimizing the effects on the woman's body.

Natural cycle IVF uses the woman's own cycle under sophisticated scanning techniques and the egg is collected before it would naturally be released. It is then fertilized in vitro and replaced back into the uterus as in standard IVF.

http://www.telegraph.co.uk/health/womenshealth/7726034/A-softly-softly-approach-to-IVF-offers-women-fresh-hope.html

Undergoing IVF treatment

There is a bit of a post code lottery regarding the provision of IVF for couples having problems becoming pregnant.

> **The guideline for infertility from NICE states:**
>
> In women aged under 40 years who have not conceived after 2 years of regular unprotected intercourse or 12 cycles of artificial insemination (where 6 or more are by intrauterine insemination), offer 3 full cycles of IVF, with or without ICSI. If the woman reaches the age of 40 during treatment, complete the current full cycle but do not offer further full cycles.
>
> **National Institute for Health and Care Excellence (2013) Adapted from CG 156 Fertility: assessment and treatment for people with fertility problems. Manchester: NICE. Available from www.nice.org.uk/CG156 Reproduced with permission.**

> In women aged 40–42 years who have not conceived after 2 years of regular unprotected intercourse or 12 cycles of artificial insemination (where 6 or more are by intrauterine insemination), offer 1 full cycle of IVF, with or without ICSI, provided the following 3 criteria are fulfilled:
>
> - they have never previously had IVF treatment
> - there is no evidence of low ovarian reserve
> - there has been a discussion of the additional implications of IVF and pregnancy at this age.
>
> **National Institute for Health and Care Excellence (2013) Adapted from CG 156 Fertility: assessment and treatment for people with fertility problems. Manchester: NICE. Available from www.nice.org.uk/CG156 Reproduced with permission.**

But it is not necessarily the case that the treatment recommended in the NICE guidelines is what will be offered for free on the NHS. It is rather dependent on the individual Clinical Commissioning Group (CCG) the couple is registered under. There are other limitations to this as well; for example, having other children lowers the potential for NHS treatment.

Implementation of these guidelines is still occurring across England, meaning the number of fertility treatment cycles you can receive on the NHS varies from region to region.

Decision making on the amount of funding is made at a local level by Clinical Commissioning Groups. Some Clinical Commissioning Groups in England fund one cycle, some two, and others the full three cycles. There are a few Clinical Commissioning Groups who do not fund IVF or ICSI at all.

The Department of Health has said that all Clinical Commissioning Groups, in the long term, should provide the full three cycles of IVF as set out in the NICE guidelines.

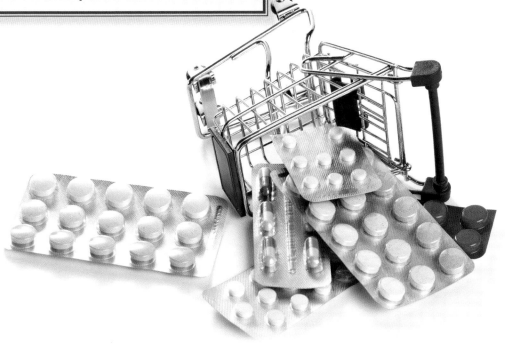

Access to funding

PCTs across England have different eligibility criteria for access to funding. These can include:

- limits on a patient's BMI (Body Mass Index - a measurement of obesity)

- whether or not the patient already has children

- the number of previous fertility treatment cycles taken.

http://www.hfea.gov.uk/fertility-treatment-cost-nhs.html

Approximately 40% of all infertility treatments are paid for by the NHS, with 60% being privately funded. While there may be fewer choices as to where the couple can go for NHS funded treatments, there will be more choice for privately funded ones and there are differences in cost and effectiveness of these clinics. There is a list of registered clinics on the Human Fertilisation and Embryology Authority (HFEA) website and local clinics can be searched for. On this list each clinic provides a breakdown of the statistics achieved regarding live births per treatment so it is possible to do a comparison.

http://guide.hfea.gov.uk/guide/

Depending upon the age of the female and the clinic, there may be a one in three or one in four possibility of pregnancy, dropping to much lower in the more mature woman. It is worth remembering that a 1/3 (33%) live baby rate is equivalent to one in three cycles resulting in a baby. This means that two of the three cycles will fail.

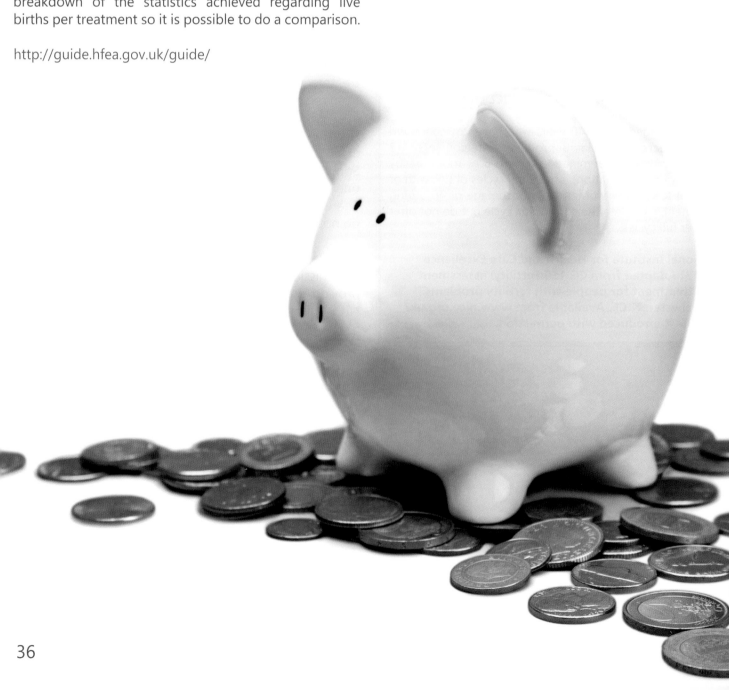

Other potential avenues

Remember that reflexology is a holistic therapy and there may well be lifestyle changes that the client can make (both male and female!) that will increase their chance of conceiving. There are some changes that are backed by evidence and some changes that are only supported by anecdotal evidence.

The National Institute For Health and Care Excellence (NICE) Guideline for Fertility and Conception

Who are NICE?

NICE's role is to improve outcomes for people using the NHS and other public health and social care services. We do this by:

- * **Producing** evidence based guidance and advice for health, public health and social care practitioners.*

- * **Developing** quality standards and performance metrics for those providing and commissioning health, public health and social care services.*

- * **Providing** a range of informational services for commissioners, practitioners and managers across the spectrum of health and social care.*

https://www.nice.org.uk/about/what-we-do

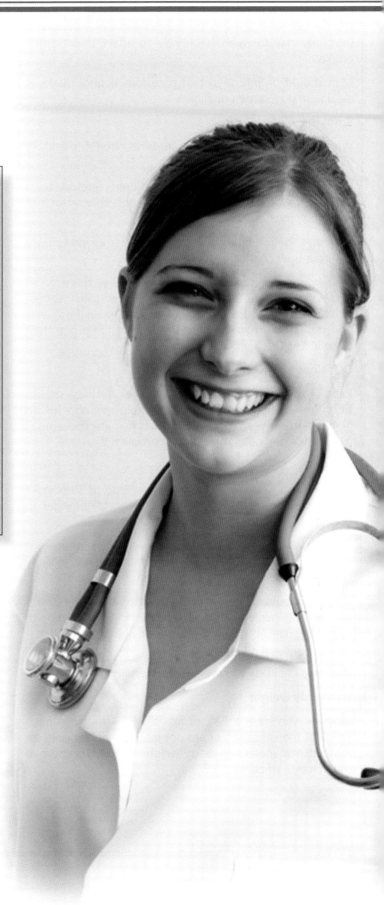

NICE Guidelines for Fertility and Conception

Alcohol

Women who are trying to become pregnant should be informed that drinking no more than 1 or 2 units of alcohol once or twice per week and avoiding episodes of intoxication reduces the risk of harming a developing fetus.

Men should be informed that alcohol consumption within the Department of Health's recommendations of 3 to 4 units per day for men is unlikely to affect their semen quality.

Men should be informed that excessive alcohol intake is detrimental to semen quality.

Smoking

Women who smoke should be informed that this is likely to reduce their fertility.

Women who smoke should be offered referral to a smoking cessation programme to support their efforts in stopping smoking.

Women should be informed that passive smoking is likely to affect their chance of conceiving.

Men who smoke should be informed that there is an association between smoking and reduced semen quality (although the impact of this on male fertility is uncertain), and that stopping smoking will improve their general health.

Caffeinated beverages

People who are concerned about their fertility should be informed that there is no consistent evidence of an association between consumption of caffeinated beverages (tea, coffee and colas) and fertility problems*.

Obesity

Women who have a body mass index (BMI) of 30 or over should be informed that they are likely to take longer to conceive.

Women who have a BMI of 30 or over and who are not ovulating should be informed that losing weight is likely to increase their chance of conception.

Women should be informed that participating in a group programme involving exercise and dietary advice leads to more pregnancies than weight loss advice alone.

Men who have a BMI of 30 or over should be informed that they are likely to have reduced fertility.

Low body weight

Women who have a BMI of less than 19 and who have irregular menstruation or are not menstruating should be advised that increasing body weight is likely to improve their chance of conception.

Tight underwear

Men should be informed that there is an association between elevated scrotal temperature and reduced semen quality, but that it is uncertain whether wearing loose-fitting underwear improves fertility

Occupation

Some occupations involve exposure to hazards that can reduce male or female fertility and therefore a specific enquiry about occupation should be made to people who are concerned about their fertility and appropriate advice should be offered.

Prescribed, over-the-counter and recreational drug use

A number of prescription, over-the-counter and recreational drugs interfere with male and female fertility, and therefore a specific enquiry about these should be made to people who are concerned about their fertility and appropriate advice should be offered.

Complementary therapy

People who are concerned about their fertility should be informed that the effectiveness of complementary therapies for fertility problems has not been properly evaluated and that further research is needed before such interventions can be recommended.

Folic acid supplementation

Women intending to become pregnant should be informed that dietary supplementation with folic acid before conception and up to 12 weeks' gestation reduces the risk of having a baby with neural tube defects. The recommended dose is 0.4 mg per day. For women who have previously had an infant with a neural tube defect or who are receiving anti-epileptic medication or who have diabetes (see Diabetes in pregnancy, NICE clinical guideline 63), a higher dose of 5 mg per day is recommended.

National Institute for Health and Care Excellence (2013) Adapted from CG 156 Fertility: assessment and treatment for people with fertility problems. Manchester: NICE. Available from www.nice.org.uk/ CG156 Reproduced with permission.

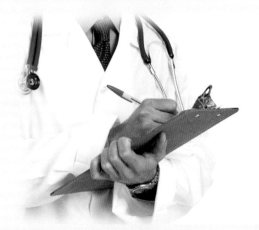

Other factors that may influence conception

If you search the internet, there is plenty of talk about what couples who are trying to conceive should and should not do; pages 37 and 38 have documented what the national guidelines say, but we will now look at some other factors which have been reported to have some benefit in conception - although evidence backing these claims may be less than scientific.

Diet

Making sure that the body provides a healthy place for a baby to grow and mature is so important for women who are looking to become pregnant. It is well understood that what we eat and drink has a direct effect on how well the body functions and may affect the chances of becoming pregnant. Eating a nutritious, well-balanced diet is a great place to start as a way to improve general health and to help maximize the chance of conception.

General diet advice for both men and women

They should:

- Eat regularly as low blood sugar levels can interfere with hormone balance.

- Cook from fresh foods and reduce the amount of 'junk food' for good nutrition.

- Eat a rainbow of food every day to ensure all minerals and vitamins are included in diet.

- Try and eat more organic food – both declining sperm count and irregular ovulation may be related to xeno-estrogens, a hormone-like chemical which is sometimes called false-oestrogen, which can interfere with hormone balance. Xeno-estrogens are found in fertilisers, pesticides and soft plastics such as cling film.

- Eat plenty of essential fatty acids that can be found in foods such as oily fish, shellfish, flaxseed (linseed), hemp oil, soya oil, rapeseed oil, pumpkin seeds, sunflower seeds, leafy vegetables and walnuts.

Some extra advice for women

Although the ovaries produce most of the oestrogen in the female body, fat cells can also make oestrogen. Some overweight women can have excess levels of the hormone and are sometimes referred to as oestrogen dominant. There is some thought that being oestrogen dominant may inhibit production of follicle-stimulating hormone (FSH) and luteinising hormone (LH), thus affecting ovulation.

Eating foods that are rich in phyto-oestrogens may help stabilize a woman's oestrogen levels as they help to prevent an excess of the real human oestrogen.

Phyto-oestrogens are found in many foods including pulses, soya, flax seed, broccoli and cabbage. A few handful-sized portions of seeds and beans and several portions of green vegetables are suggested daily.

Some extra advice for men

- Eat brazil nuts - brazil nuts are rich in selenium, a mineral that seems to help boost sperm production and improve their swimming ability. Just 2 brazil nuts a day can help produce hardier, more viable sperm cells.

- Increase vitamin C - studies have shown that increasing vitamin C intake can assist in the production of properly functioning sperm, and reduces their tendency to clump together (agglutinate). Foods rich in Vitamin C include citrus fruits. Kiwi fruits, dark green leafy vegetables, peppers etc. are all good examples of Vitamin C rich foods.

- Dark, leafy-green vegetables, such as spinach, contain high levels of folic acid. A study published in the March 2002 issue of "Fertility and Sterility" states that the combination of zinc and folic acid were found to have a positive effect in increasing sperm count and motility.

- Eat oysters, whole grains and dairy. These foods contain high levels of zinc which is effective in increasing sperm count. A study published in the "Journal of Laboratory Clinical Medicine" found that zinc deficiency in men decreased sperm count in four out of five study members. The sperm count increased as soon as the men increased their zinc intake.

(http://www.guardian.co.uk/lifeandstyle/2004/feb/15/foodanddrink.features4)

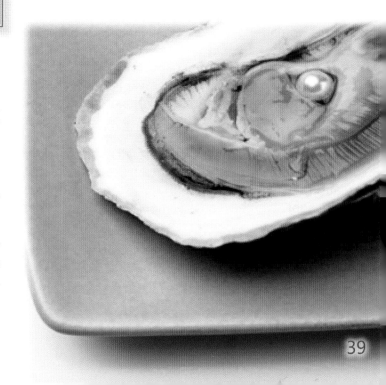

Water – the debate

Whilst everyone would agree that drinking plenty of water is essential to maintain a healthy body, there is conflicting advice as to whether tap water and/or bottled water have a role to play in infertility.

The argument against tap water is that some oestrogen excreted by women into the sewage system, is recycled back into the drinking water supply and there is concern that this may be having a detrimental effect on both male and female fertility.

The argument about water in plastic bottles is that the plastic contains a chemical called Bisphenol A (BPA) which transfers into the water, but only in tiny amounts. BPA has been accused of causing health problems such as infertility and miscarriage. Currently, there is only evidence that it can cause these problems in mice, and there is no evidence in humans. At this time, scientists are "suspicious" but can't prove its effect.

Caffeine

Reducing caffeine is not something that the NICE guidelines recognise as necessary. The research on whether caffeine can affect fertility is, however, mixed. Experts generally agree that low to moderate caffeine consumption (less than two mugs of coffee per day) won't get in the way of getting pregnant.

However, if your client is having difficulty conceiving or is undergoing in vitro fertilization, some fertility specialists say that caffeine should be avoided due to the fact that caffeine can constrict blood vessels and may slow blood flow to the uterus, thus potentially making it harder for an egg to implant.

Healthy weight

Being a healthy weight when starting to try for a baby is also important. Being overweight may make a woman oestrogen dominant and they are more likely to suffer from menstrual irregularities (see phyto-oestrogens on page 39). This is due to fat cells producing more oestrogen, which can interrupt the menstrual cycle. Women with a BMI of more than 35 can take twice as long to conceive. Being underweight can cause even greater problems; a woman needs at least 18% body fat to ovulate. If their body weight falls below this, ovulation may be disrupted or stop altogether. Underweight women, on average, take four times longer to conceive.

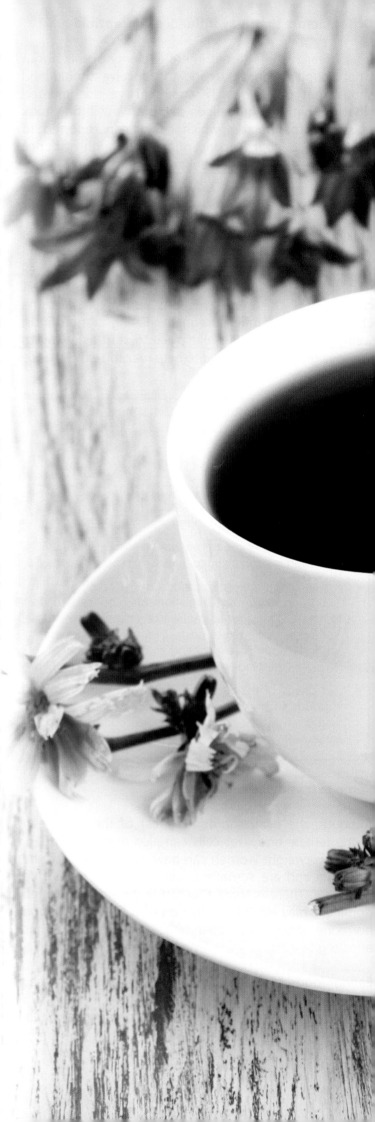

If the woman needs to either put on weight or lose weight, this should be done slowly by adopting a regular, healthy eating pattern.

Keep a cool scrotum!

The whole process of sperm production takes 64 days and is very sensitive to changes in temperature, hormones and illness. The optimal temperature in men is two degrees below body temperature; therefore periods of raised temperature (for example a fever) can have a negative effect on sperm quality. The NICE guidelines talk about not wearing tight underwear or trousers, but there are other lifestyle factors that can also cause the scrotum to become too warm, which will impair the production of healthy sperm:

- Cycling has been associated with poor sperm quality, and men should avoid cycling for long periods.

- Laptops should not be used on the lap as they generate heat.

- Sitting for long periods can also cause the testicles to be pushed too far into the body and therefore they can become too warm. Men who sit for long periods should be encouraged to get up and move around at least once an hour.

- Some people also believe that mobile phones should not be kept in trouser pockets.

- Jobs may have an impact. According to Gordon Ramsay, many chefs have low sperm counts as they are standing against hot ovens for much of the day!

Exercise

Both males and females should be encouraged to take moderate exercise. The recommended exercise at present is 30 minutes five times a week. Exercise helps maintain a healthy body. However, extreme exercise should not be undertaken by couples who are trying to conceive as this has been associated with reduced fertility in both men and women.

Stress

This will be covered in more detail in the next section. However, it is important to emphasise that high stress levels can affect fertility and that people wishing to conceive need to build time into their busy lives for relaxation.

Foresight - the Association for the promotion of pre-conceptual care

Foresight is a registered charity (http://www.foresight-preconception.org.uk).

They state that they have "put together a thoroughly researched pre-conception programme which addresses all the key infertility areas of concern in prospective parents".

They use hair analysis and state that "Foresight has been testing hair and giving supplement programmes to restore natural fertility and ensure successful reproduction for over 30 years".

They analyse the hair to look for minerals that are missing and to look for toxins in the body such as heavy metals. They will then put an individualized programme together which may include supplements, as well as advice about changes that need to be made to the environment, and dietary advice.

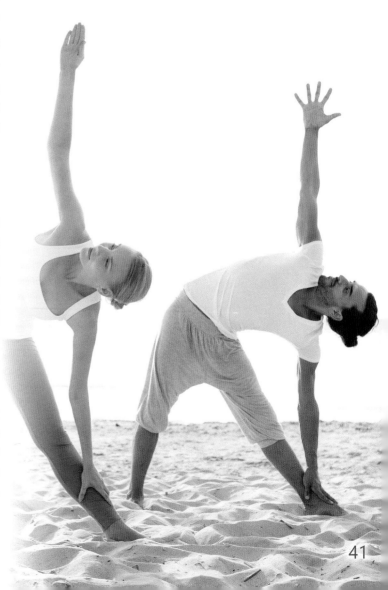

What can I, as a reflexologist, recommend to a client?

As a reflexologist, you are allowed to give general lifestyle advice to clients, including advice on general diet, water intake, alcohol consumption, smoking, exercise, sleep etc.

No unqualified advice should be given. You may not recommend any supplements, herbal remedies, aromatherapy, over the counter medications, etc. unless you are qualified to do so. These all fall out of the scope of practice as a reflexologist.

Being able to give advice starts with taking a full case history from clients. There is no point just giving out general advice i.e. drink plenty of water, take regular exercise, eat 5 portions of fruit and vegetables a day etc. – because they may already be doing this. All advice needs to be specific to the client that is sitting in front of you.

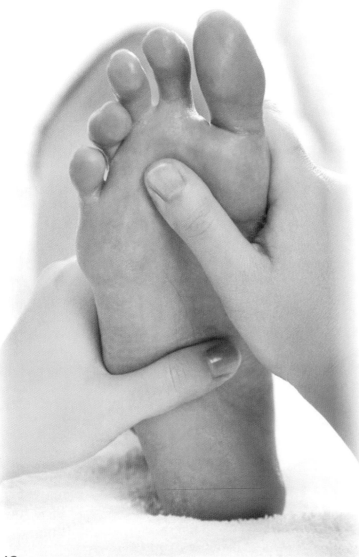

When you see a client who is trying to conceive make sure you take a full history, including information on the following:

1. Alcohol consumption.

2. Smoking and recreational drugs.

3. Caffeine intake.

4. Diet:

    a) How regular are meals?

    b) Fresh food or 'ready meals'?

    c) Variety of food – aim for a rainbow every day.

5. Water intake – and whether it is bottled, tap or filtered.

6. Exercise – how long and how often?

7. Competitiveness – are they very competitive? This can have an effect on hormone levels.

8. Assess if you consider they are overweight or underweight.

9. Stress levels and how they relax.

10. Are they taking any medications?

    a) Prescribed - have they discussed with their doctor if these are likely to interfere with fertility?

    b) Over the counter – have they checked with the pharmacist if these are likely to interfere with fertility?

11. Men – discuss lifestyle regarding keeping the scrotum cool:

    a) Tight underwear.

    b) Cycling.

    c) Laptops.

    d) Sitting.

12. Have they received any counselling or attended any fertility support groups?

You then need to consider what area of their lifestyle may be affecting their fertility (if any). Reflect back on the information in this chapter and look for any areas that they could change. This can then be offered as specific advice for them as an individual.

A word about competitiveness

The need for victory and the defeat if it happens causes testosterone levels in both men and women to rise and fall. Also, in defeat, cortisol levels rise rather similarly to when the individual is stressed. If your client is highly competitive, ask them to try a different, less competitive sport like swimming. But explain that even swimming against a time or always needing to do better can be competitive in itself.

http://www.ncbi.nlm.nih.gov/pubmed/22429747

If there are many areas that you feel need to be changed, it is important that you do not ask them to change too much at one time. They may feel daunted and feel they will fail, and will consequently ask why they should change anything.

Look back at the evidence and start with factors where there is good evidence i.e. smoking, alcohol, body weight, too much heat on the scrotum, etc.

Discuss with them what they feel is achievable; they may not feel able to give up smoking altogether but may be happy to try and reduce the number of cigarettes they are smoking. Set small, achievable goals so they feel proud that they have achieved them. They are much more likely to make changes if they feel they have been involved in the decision.

As time progresses and changes are made you can then begin to introduce new ideas that have less evidence backing them such as organic foods, caffeine etc.

Remember: always praise any change that they make, however small it is!

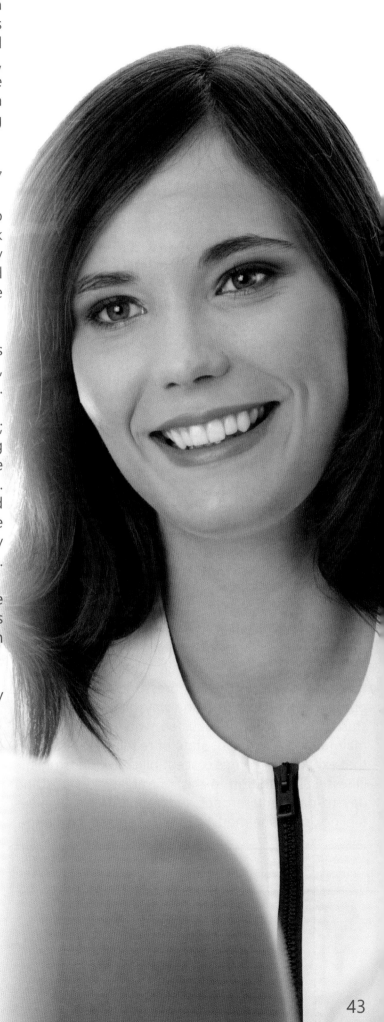

Stress and infertility

Stress is a complex condition which affects almost all parts of the body in some way. There is also some evidence to suggest that it may affect fertility. Cortisol is a hormone released in response to stress that can cause the release of an inhibiting hormone, which reduces the production of follicle stimulating hormone and luteinising hormone. Both of these hormones are integral to the release of the egg and the implantation of embryo after fertilisation. In other words, feeling stressed may be detrimental to the chances of achieving a successful pregnancy.

G.M. Buck Louis, K.J. Lum, M.S. Rajeshwari Sundaram, Z. Chen, S. Kim, C.D. Lynch, E.F Schisterman, C. Pyper (2010) Stress reduces conception probabilities across the fertile window: evidence in support of relaxation. In Fertility and Sterility Vol 95, No 7, pp 2184 – 2189

What is stress?

The most widely used definition of stress says that stress is a condition that occurs when a person perceives that "demands exceed the personal and social resources the individual is able to mobilize". According to the Oxford dictionary, stress is "a state of mental or emotional strain or tension resulting from adverse or demanding circumstances" – in other words, stress is what happens to the body when the level of pressure it is feeling goes beyond its natural ability to cope with it. When this happens, the body's response to pressure goes beyond preparing the body to run away or fight; the body starts to become exhausted with the effort of maintaining a constant state of readiness – and with that exhaustion comes susceptibility to opportunistic illnesses. In addition to this, our ability to withstand day-to-day stimuli erodes, and we might find ourselves feeling overwhelmed at the slightest challenge.

Lazarus R.S. (1966), Psychological stress and the coping process, New York: McGraw-Hill

Another way of expressing this is to look at the three stages of stress as defined by Hans Selye (1907-1982), a Hungarian endocrinologist, who was the first to give a scientific explanation for biological stress. His model states that an event that threatens an organism's well-being (a stressor) leads to a three-stage bodily response:

- **Stage 1: Alarm**
  - Upon encountering a stressor, the body reacts with the "fight-or-flight" response and the sympathetic nervous system is activated.
  - Hormones such as cortisol and adrenalin are released into the bloodstream to meet the threat or danger.
  - The body's resources are ready for "fight-or-flight".

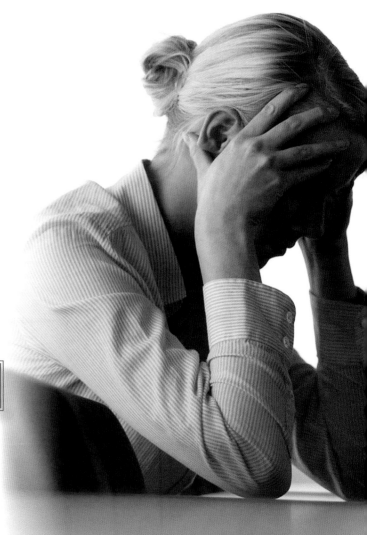

Stage 2: Resistance

➤ The parasympathetic nervous system returns many physiological functions to normal levels while the body focuses resources against the stressor.

➤ Blood glucose levels remain high; cortisol and adrenalin continue to circulate at elevated levels, but the outward appearance of the organism seems normal.

➤ Heart Rate, Blood Pressure and breathing remain rapid.

➤ The body remains on alert.

• Stage 3: Exhaustion

If the stressor continues beyond the body's capacity to cope with it, the organism exhausts resources and becomes susceptible to disease and death.

Although cortisol is essential for providing energy in the alarm stage, if the stressor continues and the person heads into the resistance and then on to the exhaustion phase, the increased cortisol level has an effect on long term non-essential requirements; it decreases the immune system and the inflammatory response. It also suppresses the digestive and reproductive systems, reduces thyroid function and heightens sugar uptake.

For further reading on stress, the AoR have produced a booklet called Stress: a Reflexologist's Guide which is available to buy via the website (www.aor.org.uk).

Does infertility cause stress, anxiety and depression?

Trying for a baby in itself can be an extremely stressful event - especially when it has taken longer than expected. You will see, or will have seen, this for yourself; women who are trying to conceive often display symptoms of anxiety and/or depression and the longer they have been trying, the greater the distress can become.

"Women who experience infertility are more likely to suffer from heightened depression and anxiety symptoms than women in general. The longer the infertility and the greater the associated distress, the more likely a patient will suffer

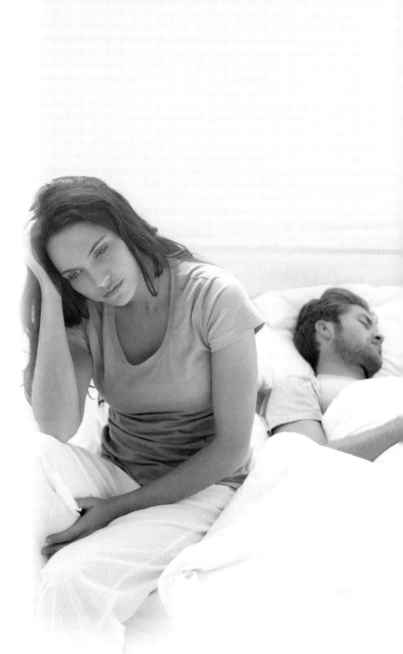

depressive symptoms, which can in turn diminish fertility and interfere with treatment success."

(http://www.iaac.ca/content/stress-and-distress-in-fertility-dr-alice-domar-spring-2010)

A study also showed that stress levels of infertile women can be equivalent to women with cancer, AIDS, or heart disease.

(http://www.psychologytoday.com/blog/when-youre-not-expecting/201103/the-stress-trying-get-pregnant).

Many women feel that if they have not conceived, they cannot be a true woman (even if the problem lies with the male) and they feel like a failure. There is also the worry about leaving a legacy; by having a child you know you will leave part of yourself behind when you die, so if you are unable to have a child, how will you be remembered?

There are many studies which have identified that the anxiety and depression that can result from long term stress is a real issue for women who are trying to conceive (interestingly, there appears to be no research for men). These include: Women who experience infertility report significantly higher levels of depressive symptoms (1) and anxiety (2) than women in the fertile population. In one study, 11% of infertile women met the criteria for a major depressive episode, compared to 3.6% of fertile women (3). A study of infertile women found that half of the subjects reported changes in their sexual function, and 75% reported changes in mood, such as increased feelings of sadness (2).

(1) Domar AD, Broome A, Zuttermeister PC, et al. The prevalence and predictability of depression in infertile women. Fertil Steril 1992; 58:1158-63.
(2) Downey J, Yinling S, McKinney M, et al. Mood disorders, psychiatric symptoms, and distress in women presenting for infertility evaluation. Fertil Steril 1989; 52:425-32.
(3) Downey J, McKinney M. The psychiatric status of women presenting for infertility evaluation. Am J Orthopsych 1992; 62:196-205.

"The impact of stress on conception has been under debate for a number of years. In the 60's women were often advised to "just relax," or to "take a second honeymoon," which felt infuriating, especially when it moved the responsibility from the physician to the woman. Furthermore, since about half of infertility is due to a male factor, women resented being targeted as needing to monitor their stress levels. Ultimately, as physicians were able more clearly to diagnose physiological causes for a couple's infertility, the "relax" advice diminished and assisted reproductive technologies claimed increasing credit for success rates in conception. So, even as folk wisdom may have promoted stress as a cause of infertility, physicians tended to agree that stress, when it was present, was most likely to be an effect of infertility."

(http://www.psychologytoday.com/blog/when-youre-not-expecting/201103/the-stress-trying-get-pregnant)

As a reflexologist, it is therefore essential that when you are preparing a client for conception, you need to be aware that there may well be underlying distress, anxiety and/or depression. Allow your client time to express how they are feeling; you may also feel they should seek help, and they should be able to arrange counselling through their GP.

Does stress affect fertility?

The reproductive system is seen by the body as irrelevant in the stress response. This means that blood supply to the organs of the reproductive system becomes restricted as the blood is directed to those organs directly concerned with fight or flight, which can lead to malfunction of the reproductive organs. A long term stress response can lead to erectile dysfunction in men and an impaired lubrication function in women, as well as a reduction in sexual desire through lack of blood supply to the higher order parts of the brain which contribute to sexual desire.

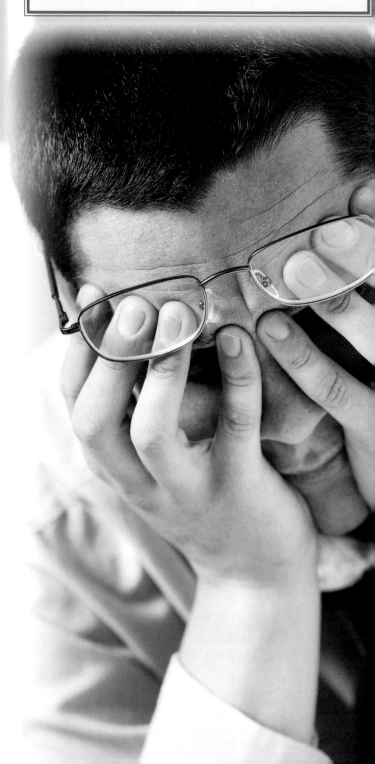

We already know that stress is a complex condition which affects almost all parts of the body in some way and there is some evidence to suggest that it may affect fertility. It is hypothesised that the mechanical link between stress and fertility is mainly an endocrine one. It starts in the hypothalamus, which communicates between the nervous system and the endocrine system. The hypothalamus secretes a range of hormones. One of these hormones is called gonadotrophic-releasing hormone (GnRH) which passes into the anterior lobe of the pituitary gland to stimulate the release of two further hormones:

- Luteinising hormone (LH), which prepares the lining of the uterus to receive an embryo.

- Follicle stimulating hormone (FSH), which stimulates the ovaries to release an ovum (egg) into the fallopian tube.

When a person is stressed, the hypothalamus secretes a substance called corticotrophin releasing factor, which is a neurotransmitter that passes from the hypothalamus to the pituitary. This stimulates the anterior part of the pituitary gland to produce adrenocorticotrophic hormone (ACTH). This is a message-carrying hormone which passes through the blood stream to stimulate the adrenal glands. In response to this hormone, the adrenal glands begin to produce adrenalin, noradrenalin and cortisol.

It is suggested that glucocorticoids (a group of hormones including cortisol, which are associated with the stress response) stimulate the release of a hormone known as gonadotrophin-inhibitory hormone (GnIH), which suppresses the production of GnRH in the hypothalamus. GnIH suppresses the production of FSH and LH.

In a woman, this would mean that there would be less of a chance of her releasing an ovum to be fertilised in the first place – and it may also mean that even if the ovum is fertilised, the uterus may not be fully prepared to receive the embryo. This may lessen the likelihood of the pregnancy progressing beyond fertilisation, as the embryo would not be able to embed in the endometrium (uterine lining) and begin to grow.

Moberg, G.P, (1987) Influence of the adrenal axis upon the gonads. In Clarke, J.R, (ed), Oxford Reviews of Reproductive Biology, Vol. 9. Clarendon Press, Oxford, pp 456 – 496.

S.L. Berga, T.L. Davies and D.E. Giles (1997) Women with functional hypothalamic amenorrhea but not other forms of anovulation display amplified cortisol concentrations. In Fertility and Sterility Vol 67 No. 6, pp 1024 – 1030

M.D. Marcus, T.L. Loucks, S.L.Berga (2001) Psychological correlates of functional hypothalamic amenorrhea. In Fertility and Sterility Vol 76 No. 2, pp310 – 316

K.A. Sanders and N.W. Bruce (1997) A prospective study of psychosocial stress and fertility. In Human Reproduction Vol 12 No. 10, pp2324 – 2329

G.M. Buck Louis, K.J. Lum, M.S. Rajeshwari Sundaram, Z. Chen, S. Kim, C.D. Lynch, E.F Schisterman, C. Pyper (2010) Stress reduces conception probabilities across the fertile window: evidence in support of relaxation. In Fertility and Sterility Vol 95, No 7, pp 2184 – 2189

E.D. Kirby, A.C. Geraghty, T. Ubuka, G.E. Bentley and D. Kaufer (2009) Stress increases putative gonadotrophin inhibitory hormone and decreases luteinizing hormone in male rats. In PNAS Vol 106 No. 27, pp 11324 - 11329

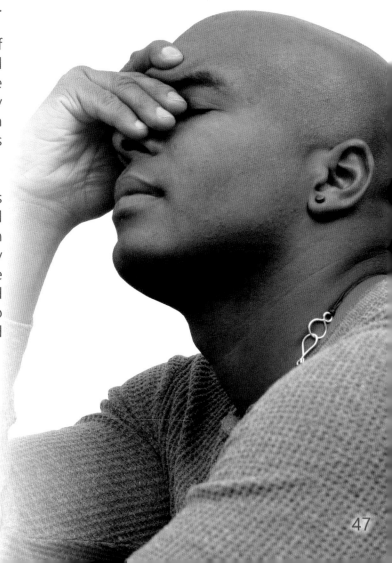

There are some other research papers that back these findings up:

- Stress significantly reduces the probability of conception each day during the fertile window.

G.M. Buck Louis, K.J. Lum, M.S. Rajeshwari Sundaram, Z. Chen, S. Kim, C.D. Lynch, E.F Schisterman, C. Pyper (2010) Stress reduces conception probabilities across the fertile window: evidence in support of relaxation. In Fertility and Sterility Vol 95, No 7, pp 2184 – 2189

- Depressive symptoms are associated with decreased fertility and can interfere with the success of infertility treatment. In one investigation, women with a lifetime history of clinical depression were nearly twice as likely to report infertility as those not depressed.

Lapane LK, Zierler S, Lasatar TM, et al. Is a history of depressive symptoms associated with an increased risk of infertility in women? Psychosom Med 1995; 57(6):509-13

- In vitro fertilization (IVF) patients who reported heightened levels of depressive symptoms prior to beginning IVF treatment had significantly lower success rates than women with lower levels of depressive symptoms.

Thiering P, Beaurepaire J, Jones M, et al. Mood state as a predictor of treatment outcome after in vitro fertilization/ embryo transfer technology. J Psychosom Res 1993; 37:481-91.

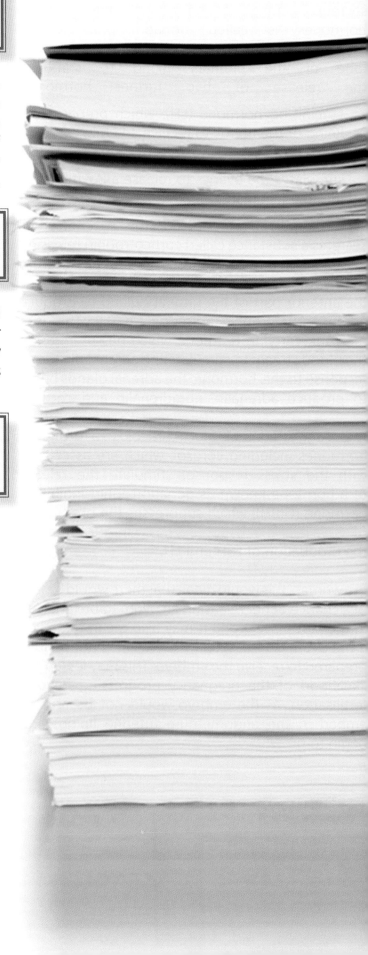

The effect of spirituality on fertility

Dr Alice Dorman also discusses the impact that spiritual wellbeing has on stress levels. In an evaluation of nearly 200 infertile women, high levels of religiosity and spirituality are significantly correlated with low levels of psychological distress. "A high level of spiritual wellbeing is significantly linked with less infertility distress and fewer depressive symptoms, suggesting a relationship between spirituality and the psychological wellbeing of women undergoing infertility treatment. Conversely, self-reported depressive symptoms and lower levels of spiritual wellbeing predict higher levels of infertility distress. Spirituality and religion are important sources of solace for most individuals."

(http://www.iaac.ca/content/stress-and-distress-infertility-dr-alice-domar-spring-2010)

Even if you do not consider yourself to be religious or you feel uncomfortable discussing the spiritual side of things, it may be of value to enquire about and support patients' religious beliefs to help promote their physical and psychological wellbeing, in order to help maximise their fertility. You could simply ask, "do you have any religious or spiritual beliefs?" This will allow them a window to talk about it if they wish. You are not there to preach, just to listen and be non-judgmental.

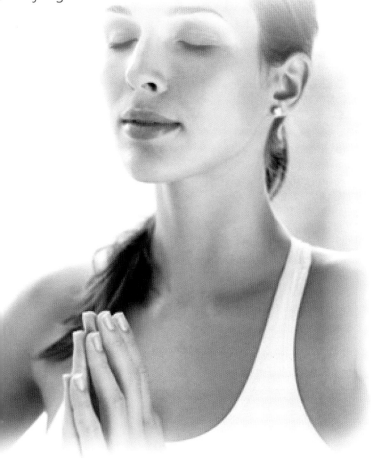

Can reflexology help reduce stress?

There appears to be good evidence that infertility can cause stress and stress can cause infertility. This can become a vicious downward spiral, and the best way to break this spiral is surely to try and aid relaxation and reduce stress levels; reflexology is one way of doing this.

"We are left with the awareness that many women would do anything to be rid of the stress that accompanies their infertility. So, whether or not stress can be credibly shown to be associated with fertility failure, women being treated for infertility should be offered every opportunity, with their partners, to participate in mind-body workshops and other forms of relaxation that can diminish their stress."

> The Stress of Trying to Get Pregnant. Published on March 4, 2011 by Connie Shapiro, PhD in When You're Not Expecting

Stress is particularly important because we are being restricted in what we can say, courtesy of the Advertising Standards Authority. However, they do let us say that reflexology:

- helps relax
- improves mood
- aids sleep
- helps relieve tension
- improves a sense of wellbeing

So this is a prime example of where we can celebrate the fact that reflexology has been shown to affect the above, and for couples who are trying to conceive, these benefits could make a difference to their fertility.

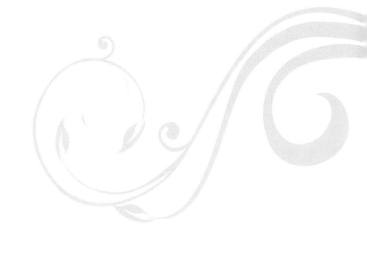

Some of the studies that have allowed us to use the phrases shown on the previous page include the references below:

- Holt et al 2009 showed that while it was an underpowered trial of anovulatory women and reflexology which was not able to provide clear evidence for the clinical use of reflexology, there was a significant decrease in the Hospital Anxiety and Depression scale ratings in the active group. No such response was seen in the sham reflexology group. Its last sentence states that 'Future studies should consider exploring the relationship between reflexology and depression.' (1)

- McVicar et al 2007, were validating a measure of anxiety for use in cancer patients receiving reflexology. But it was initially used in healthy individuals as a test of methodology and although these individuals were not exhibiting clinical anxiety there was still a statistically significant reduction in their anxiety state after reflexology. (2)

- A small study of breast and lung cancer patients showed a significant decrease in anxiety after reflexology. (3)

- A larger randomised controlled trial of reflexology and the psychological effects in early breast cancer patients, showed that reflexology has a statistically significant and clinically worthwhile effect on quality of life (QoL), which includes anxiety and stress levels. (4)

- Two audits of cancer patients' perceptions of reflexology (5) resulted in an 'increased ability to cope with side effects' and 'time out' from their illness. In well yet stressed individuals, this increased ability to cope and time out could well be important with coping with the day to day demands of life. A second result was, again, improved quality of life, relief of symptoms and of psychological and spiritual distress. (6)

- A small study on patients with neurological illnesses included 33 post treatment comments about feeling calmer and less tense. There was also a statistical drop in systolic blood pressure and heart rate. (7)

- A small study looked at two NHS healthcare trusts that held stress awareness days; these included 'taster' sessions of reflexology and other therapies. 75% of attendees believed they had benefited from attending. (8)

References:

(1) The effectiveness of foot reflexology in inducing ovulation: a sham-controlled randomized trial Jane Holt, Jonathan Lord, Umesh Acharya, Adrian White, Nyree O'Neill, Steve Shaw, Andy Barton Fertility and Sterility, Vol. 91, Issue 6, p2514–2519

(2) Evaluation of anxiety, salivary cortisol and melatonin secretion following reflexology treatment: A pilot study in healthy individuals, A.J. Mc Vicar, C.R. Greenwood, F. Fewell, V. D'Arcy, S. Chandrasekharan and L.C. Alldridge. Complementary Therapies in Clinical Practice, 2007 VOL 13; NUMBER 3, page(s) 137-145

(3) The Effects of Foot Reflexology on Anxiety and Pain in Patients With Breast and Lung Cancer Stephenson, N. L. Weinrich, S. P. Tavakolil, A. S. ONCOLOGY NURSING FORUM 2000 VOL 27; PART 1 , page(s) 67-76

(4) A randomised, controlled trial of the psychological effects of reflexology in early breast cancer Donald M. Sharp, Mary B. Walker, Amulya Chaturvedi, Sunil Upadhyay, Abdel Hamid, Andrew A. Walker, Julie S. Bateman, Fiona Braid, Karen Ellwood, Claire Hebblewhite, Teresa Hope, Michael Lines, Leslie G. Walker European Journal of cancer 2010 VOL 46; NUMBER 2, page(s) 312-322

(5) Evaluation of a hospice based reflexology service: a qualitative audit of patient perceptions Gambles, M. Crooke, M. Wilkinson, S. EUROPEAN JOURNAL OF ONCOLOGY NURSING 2002 VOL 6; NUMB 1, page(s) 37-44

(6) Reflexology audit: patient satisfaction, impact on quality of life and availability in Scottish hospices Milligan, M Fanning, M. Hunter, S. Tadjali, M. Stevens, E. INTERNATIONAL JOURNAL OF PALLIATIVE NURSING 2002 VOL 8; PART 10 , page(s) 489-496

(7) Just the ticket': integrating massage and reflexology in practice (part 2) Dryden, S. L. Holden, S. D. Mackereth, P. A. COMPLEMENTARY THERAPIES IN NURSING AND MIDWIFERY Complementary Therapies in Nursing and Midwifery 1999 5, 19-21

(8) Would complementary and alternative medicine be welcome in the workplace? R.Philipp, P. Thorne. Public health 2008 Vol 122, issue 10, 1124 – 1127

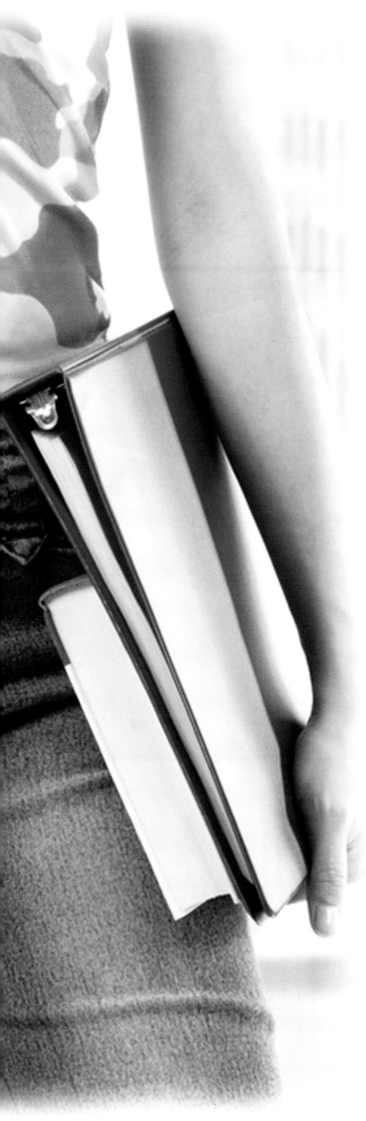

A research study to be aware of

You need to be aware of the study below and its faults in case you are ever faced with this as a reason to not advise reflexology.

A study was published in 2009, the results of which showed that "the use of complementary and alternative medicine (CAM) therapies during treatment with Assisted Reproduction Technique (ART) was associated with a 30% lower pregnancy and live birth rate."

This study has, however, been heavily criticized in the medical and complementary therapy press. The study was an observational study that looked at individuals who were spontaneous users and non-users (i.e. those that had themselves chosen to have a CAM therapy and those that had not). The researchers then compared on-going pregnancies and live birth rates over a 12 month period of ART.

The main issue with the study was that at the start of the trial, the information collected was only about demographics (e.g. age, years married) and medical information (e.g. years infertile, whether they already have children) as well as information about the number of and types of fertility treatments women had prior to study entry. There was no attempt to measure stress, anxiety or depression scores, or other psychological scores. It has been argued that those who had spontaneously sought CAM therapies may well have had higher levels of distress, which in itself would affect results.

There were also no comparisons made for different CAM therapies, therefore this offers no specific guidance for reflexology alone.

Use of complementary and alternative medicines associated with a 30% lower ongoing pregnancy/live birth rate during 12 months of fertility treatment. J. Boivin and L. Schmidt. Hum. Reprod. Advance Access published April 9, 2009. Human Reproduction, Vol.1, No.1 pp. 1–6, 2009

Self help for reducing stress levels

With ever increasing levels of stress in the world, it is important for individuals to take responsibility for their own wellbeing. Reflexology can fit into a busy lifestyle and can easily be part of an individual's coping strategy, resulting in multi-system relaxation and increased wellbeing. There are also other lifestyle changes that may help or hinder stress.

Constructive self-help methods

1. Regular complementary therapy - we recommend reflexology here. An hour of manual therapy allowing personal space may be very beneficial.

2. Regular exercise to suit the individual - for some this may be a team sport, for others something more individual like golf, dancing or yoga.

3. Reduction in stimulants - this is not just coffee; tea and most cola based drinks contain high levels of caffeine. Some energy boosting drinks are equal to multiple cups of coffee. Even chocolate contains caffeine although at lower level. Alcohol, cigarettes and recreational drugs are also all stimulants. Adding further stimulants to an already hyper-stimulated system is not helpful.

4. Healthy eating - the increase in cortisol can make you crave unhealthy foods which are high in fat, sugar and salt. Eating the right foods can help reduce the cravings and even replenish vitamins and minerals that are being depleted by the stress.

5. Doing something creative - this can be anything from drawing to sewing to singing, whatever suits the individual.

6. Increasing contact with your social relationships by visiting family and friends more.

7. Meditation or at the very least deep breathing.

8. More laughing! Smiling and laughing are thought to reduce stress levels and smiling uses fewer muscles than frowning.

9. Taking on processes to learn how to cope – for example, challenging unhelpful thoughts. There is a technique called mindfulness which is being used to treat stress, anxiety and depression. This involves using meditation and mind control to concentrate on the present, not looking backward as this cannot be changed and not

worrying about what the future may hold - why worry about something that may not happen? Jon Kabat-Zinn has written several books on the subject and developed CDs to guide the meditations.

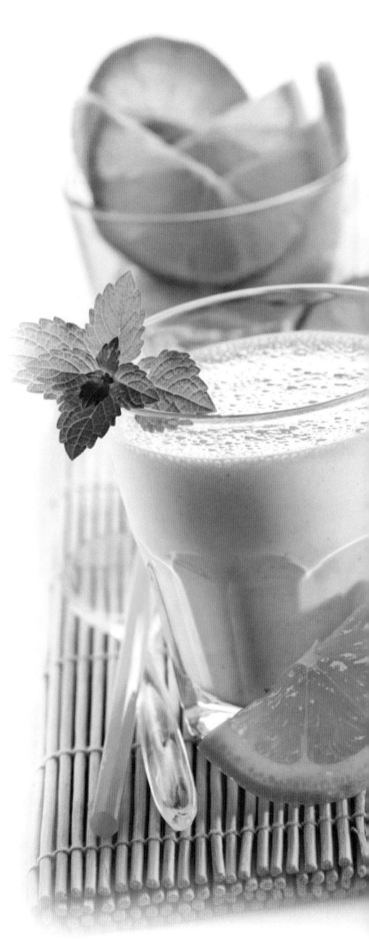

Behaviours that may add to the stress cycle

Clients should be advised that these behaviours are sometimes used in response to stress, but they only add to stress and anxiety levels and should be avoided:

1. Increased alcohol intake - the habit of one small glass of wine per night slowly increases to two large glasses.

2. Increased use of stimulants, especially recreational drugs.

3. Changes in eating patterns – eating more or less than usual.

4. Increased release of anger / frustration.

5. Lack of motivation in down time – zoning out with the TV or computer.

Summary

Do not underestimate the effect that stress has on the body including fertility; it can easily become a downward cycle of feeling bad, taking on bad habits and not being able to see a way out, which makes it all worse – and so it can go on.

It is particularly important that clients with stress are treated with an understanding, listening ear, and any advice you give regarding lifestyle changes to break this cycle must be small and achievable changes. Do not be surprised if initially they find it hard to make any changes at all; just keep talking to them and try to find a small change that they are able to make and go from there.

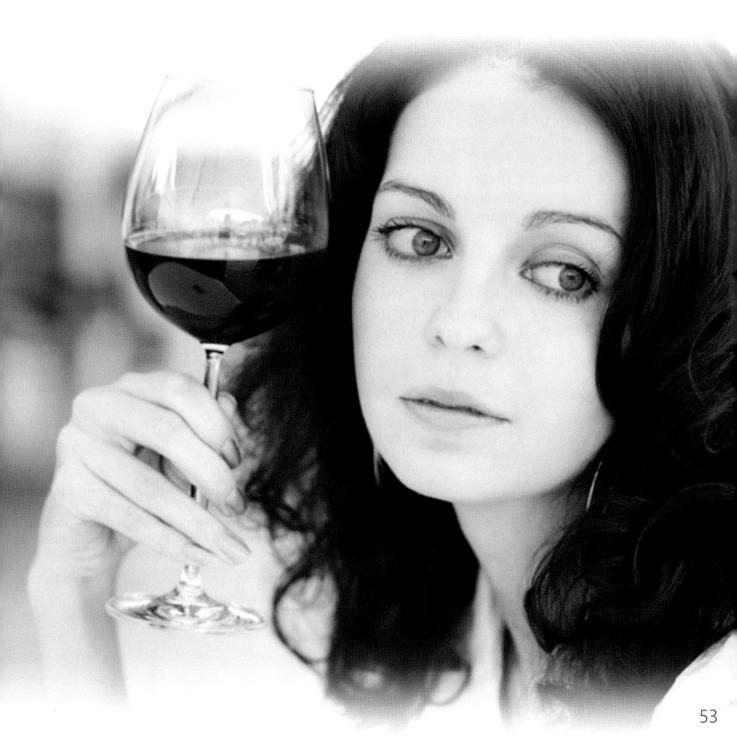

How reflexologists can help

It is important to recognise that this is a vulnerable group of women and men; they often come with high levels of stress, anxiety and depression as discussed in the last chapter. Clients will often arrive expecting reflexology to provide an instant route to conception.

Make your mantra to "under-promise and over-perform"

If you always bear in mind the above mantra and that you should (within reason of course) remain positive in your consultation (just don't make wild promises that you cannot guarantee) you run less chance of raising expectations too high. Clients are more likely to be happy with their progress, rather than being disappointed and therefore more likely to stop treatments. Be clear from the start that if they are trying for natural conception, you would like them to commit to a six month programme of reflexology to allow time for them to make lifestyle changes along the way and for the body to respond to the reflexology; hopefully this will help those that want a 'one treatment to get me pregnant' fix realise there will need to be a commitment. You will come across clients who do fall pregnant after one treatment, which is wonderful, but remember that will not be the norm for all.

For clients who are undergoing fertility treatments, you will need to adapt the reflexology timings to fit in with their treatment. This is discussed later.

Case histories

When you take a case history, you will need to take all the normal information to help identify any lifestyle changes that the client will need to make (see Other potential avenues on pages 37 - 43). However, you will need to take more information regarding their conception journey so far; this should include:

- How long have you been trying to conceive?
- Have you or your partner had any investigations?
- Do either you or your partner have children?
- Have you ever conceived before?
- Are your periods regular and when was your last period?
- Have you tried to find out when you ovulate? (optional)
- Are you having regular sexual intercourse? (this does not need to be asked on day one if you feel the client will be uncomfortable with it).
- How would you rate your stress levels?

How long have they been trying to conceive?

People who are concerned about their fertility should be informed that over 80% of couples in the general population will conceive within 1 year if:

- the woman is aged under 40 years and
- they do not use contraception and have regular sexual intercourse.

Of those who do not conceive in the first year, about half will do so in the second year (cumulative pregnancy rate over 90%). [2004, amended 2013]

National Institute for Health and Care Excellence (2013) Adapted from CG 156 Fertility: assessment and treatment for people with fertility problems. Manchester: NICE. Available from www.nice.org.uk/ CG156 Reproduced with permission.

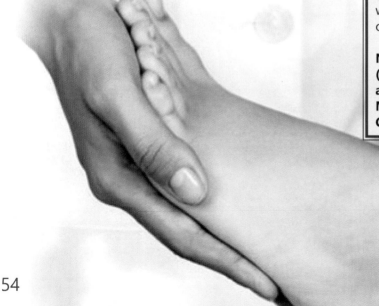

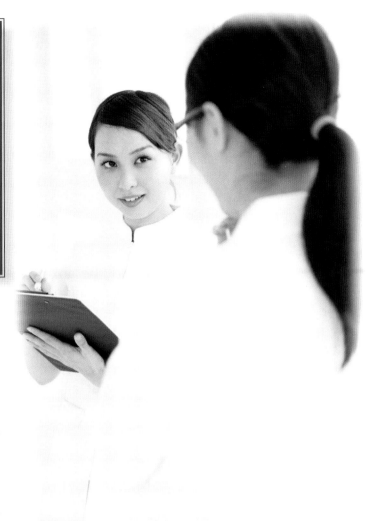

Have they or their partner had any investigations?

If your client or their partner has had investigations, this is essential information for you to know to ensure that you do not over-promise. If there is a medical reason why the couple cannot conceive, be realistic in thinking about whether reflexology could possibly change that.

We know that reflexology is a powerful therapy, but there are conditions where it would be irresponsible as a therapist to say that treatments could change the outcome. If this is the situation, clients must be encouraged to follow medical advice. Conditions where reflexology is unlikely to have an effect include: total blockage of the fallopian tubes or vas deferens, erectile dysfunction due to permanent nerve damage etc. Basically, where the problem is irreversible or there are complete blockages.

Of course, this does not mean that you cannot treat these clients - but you do need to clarify expected outcomes from the reflexology; you would be offering treatments on the basis of relaxation and general wellbeing, not to clear blockages.

Have they ever conceived before?

Although this may not give you information about how likely they are to conceive at this time, it will bring up whether they have previously carried a baby to full term or have had a miscarriage or termination; if either of the latter two are the case, there may be associated feelings of sadness or guilt that may need to be addressed. These emotions may come out in treatments or in the time between treatments and for no apparent reason. It is important to warn your client that this is positive and healing and that it will usually happen when they are feeling safe.

Are their periods regular and when was their last period?

It is important that you know if their periods are regular. If their periods are irregular, ask if they have had this investigated as there may be a known underlying cause e.g. Polycystic Ovary Syndrome (PCOS). Whatever the root cause, it will be good to work on balancing the endocrine system – some useful techniques will be discussed in the last chapter.

Let your client know that initially, it would be hoped that their periods would become more regular. Even if the client's periods are already regular, the length of the cycle might change. It is worth mentioning this so they are not alarmed if this happens.

Knowing when their last period was will let you keep a record of their cycle. It may also affect how you treat them, depending on whether they are pre or post ovulation. This will be discussed further in the next chapter 'How reflexology can help'.

Have they tried to find out when they ovulate and how often are they having sexual intercourse?

We have already talked about the best way to approach conception being to try and have regular sexual intercourse throughout the month, trying not to become obsessed with when the 'best time' is. This can increase stress and anxiety levels in both partners, as sexual intercourse can become functional rather than loving and fun.

However, you will find that many clients who come to see you for conception will already be anxious because they have been 'trying' and nothing has happened, so they may already have tried to identify when they are ovulating. I have stated that this question is optional; you do not want to put the idea that identifying the day of ovulation is essential into their head, but if they do know, it all adds to your information for treatment planning.

How would they rate their stress levels?

We have already discussed the vicious downward spiral that can occur with couples who have been trying to conceive; this can increase stress, anxiety and depression levels, which in turn can reduce the chances of conception.

It is useful to use a rating scale for stress from the first treatment onwards. This allows you to have a comparison for later on in the treatment plan and helps you check that stress levels are moving in the right direction. Perhaps use a visual analogue scale (VAS) or even a very simple 1-10 scale, and remember to keep reviewing this as treatments progress to show them how their stress levels have changed.

General lifestyle

For information on what lifestyle factors need to be looked at, refer back to *Other potential avenues* on pages 37 to 43.

Effect of reflexology on women suffering with Polycystic Ovaries (PCO) and Polycystic Ovary Syndrome (PCOS)

A pilot study was undertaken in Denmark in 2004-2005 looking at the effect that reflexology had on women who had a long cycle (33-90 days) as a result of PCO or PCOS. Eight women received 19 reflexology treatments over a 5-6 month period.

The length of their cycle significantly dropped (p=0.03) by an average of 14.81 days, and the number of follicles in the ovaries fell by an average of 16.3 follicles. There were no significant changes in hormone levels.

Although this is only a very small study, the results appear promising and there is the hope that a larger study may be carried out.

Pilot Study Indicates that Reflexology has Effect On Women Suffering from Polycystic Ovaries (PCO) and Polycystic Ovary Syndrome (PCOS). Lone Victoria Schumann, Project Manager, Bentzonsvej 9, kl.th., DK-2000 Frederiksberg.

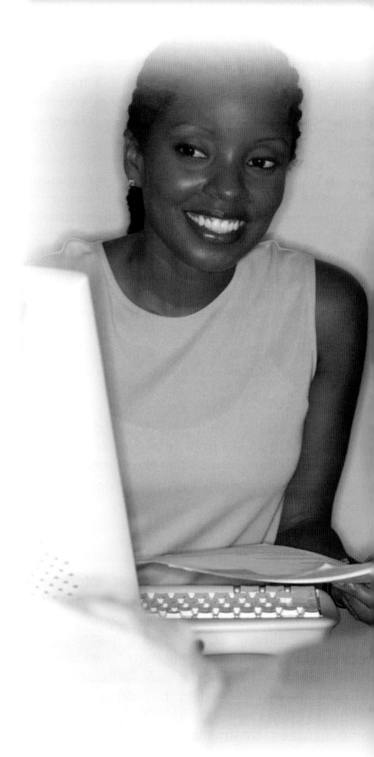

So how else can reflexologists help?

Although we are limited in what we say when we are advertising due to the Advertising Standards Authority, we are allowed to say that reflexology:

- helps relax
- improves mood
- aids sleep
- helps relieve tension
- improves a sense of wellbeing

As already stated, this is a prime example when we can celebrate the fact that reflexology has been shown to affect the above, and for couples who are trying to conceive, these benefits could make a difference to their fertility.

However, when we are actually talking to a client we can say more; but just remember to under-promise and over-perform. Yet it is also important that you adopt a positive attitude so they can begin to believe that they can conceive. When actually speaking to a client, you can use anecdotes, give examples of previous clients who you have treated with similar issues, or cases you have read about where the woman has gone on to conceive.

If this area is new to you, you will be amazed at how effective reflexology can be in relieving stress, balancing hormones and resulting in conception for women who thought they would never go on to have a baby. Believe in it yourself as this belief will transfer to your client.

Also ensure that the whole experience is focused on the client; be a listening ear if this is what they want, let them air their worries and concerns and give them time to concentrate on themselves for the hour they are with you. Having quiet time is also important during the treatment; make sure they take some time to purely relax. Clients who have been stressed for a while may have forgotten what it feels like to be relaxed; reflexology can be a start point reminding them how good it feels to be relaxed and grounded.

In these busy times, you will come across clients who spend their whole life rushing around, often feeling anxious about deadlines and pressures that they are under. If clients are feeling stressed and anxious, their hour-long reflexology treatment is only a start point for them. They need to build into their lives regular time for relaxation.

Suggest that they sit quietly a few times a week and start to think about, or visualise, how a baby will fit into their daily routines, how it will feel to hold their baby and how having a baby will change their lives. The mind is very powerful; calming it and reassuring it that there is space in their busy life to have a baby can be very beneficial.

You can also suggest that they spend at least an hour (preferably longer) each weekend reading, either reading a newspaper from cover to cover or a book. This will again help ground the client and show them that not only can they can take time off for relaxation, but how good that can feel too!

Finally, do they spend 'value' time with their partner? Clients can sometimes lose sight of the fact that their relationship still needs to be nurtured. Only spending time together to have sexual intercourse around the time of ovulation is not a normal relationship. What do they both enjoy doing together? Get them to identify this and book time in their diaries to do it! This may be a walk at the weekend, a trip to the cinema or a meal together. What they do together is not important as long as it nurtures them as a couple.

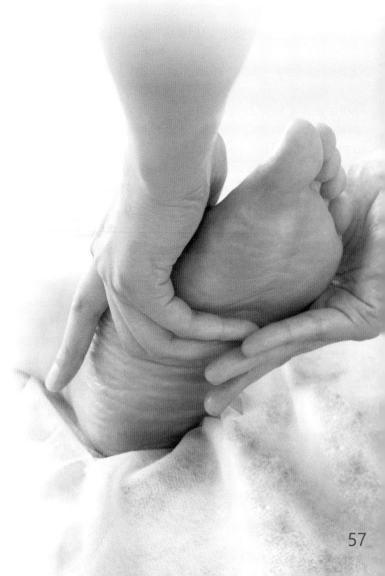

How reflexology can help
and how to adapt your treatment

There appears to be confusion and sometimes fear around when and how reflexologists should treat men and particularly woman who are trying to conceive, such as whether you should treat someone after ovulation as they may be in early stages of pregnancy without knowing it, or whether you should treat during IVF, etc. This chapter aims to guide you as to what you can do as a reflexologist and discuss when you can treat. Sometimes there is no categorical answer, so we will give you both sides of the argument for your consideration; you then need to decide which approach fits in best for you.

For the majority of clients, you will be looking to adapt your treatment to address endocrine balance or stress - or probably both. As discussed in a previous chapter, stress and infertility appear to go hand in hand, and it is wise to try and ascertain levels of stress, anxiety and depression in clients who are seeking reflexology for conception.

Reflexology – for relaxation and stress relief

There are a few basic principles that are useful to consider when you are treating clients with very high stress levels. The below advice has been adapted with kind permission from the work of Dorthe Krogsgaard HMAR and Peter Lund Frandsen HMAR, Denmark (www.touchpoint.dk):

1. With a stressed person, the physiological response has changed and it can be difficult to be "invited inside" with any kind of treatment. Therefore, pay extra attention to the initial phase of a reflexology session. Hold the feet, palms against soles, and try intuitively to feel when the connection is there. Ask the client to take 10 breaths, very slowly and quietly, breathing through the nose while you are still touching their feet. Alternatively, you can place your thumbs on the solar plexus reflexes, and ask them to take 3-10 slow breaths through their nose until your thumbs begin to sink into solar plexus, indicating that they are relaxing into your touch.

2. The entire session should be comfortable and pain free. This will help avoid increasing the sympathetic nervous system activity. It is about using a pressure that is right for your client; there needs to enough pressure that the client enjoys the sensation, but without causing pain which may add to the stress response the body is   already afflicted with.

3. It is a good idea to ask stressed clients to "leave their head" and focus on the body - especially the feet - during the treatment. Stressed people usually have so many things going on in their minds and have often lost contact with the rest of the body.

As you go along, inform your client which part of the body you are giving impulses to. Ask them to focus on the area and tell you about possible sensations or reactions in the body or in the feet.

Stressed clients are often exhausted, but in our opinion the session will be more effective if clients do not fall asleep. The energy of their consciousness or concentration seems to strengthen the healing response.

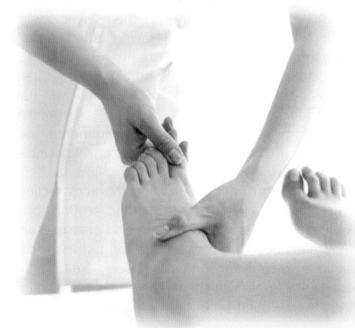

4. A stressed person needs more time for the reflexology communication process. Try to offer slow and calm impulses, and work with fewer reflexes. However, do spend more time on each reflex you treat. Make short breaks where you simply hold the feet, to allow the person to absorb the impulses.

5. Work with the autonomic nervous system (ANS), which is a key player in the stress response. One way of working with the ANS is to use the reflexes for the spinal origin of these nerves. In figure 1, the red area represents the origin of the sympathetic branch of the ANS, which is found in the lateral horn of the spinal cord in segments T1 to L2. The parasympathetic branch originates in the brain stem, upper cervical spine and sacral spine S2-S4 (blue on figure 1).

These reflexes can be worked on the plantar aspect of the foot on the periosteum of the bones (fibrous layer covering the bones) shown in the illustration. Push the soft tissue aside while working, to enable a direct contact with the bony surface.

Some reflexologists prefer to work with sedating techniques on the sympathetic branch (which is too active during chronic stress) and stimulating techniques on the parasympathetic. We may also choose to simply work all areas, letting the system adjust and find a new balance.

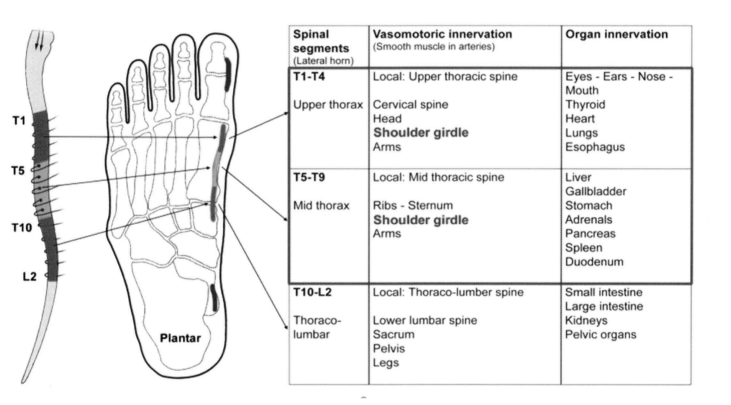

Spinal segments (Lateral horn)	Vasomotoric innervation (Smooth muscle in arteries)	Organ innervation
T1-T4 Upper thorax	Local: Upper thoracic spine Cervical spine Head **Shoulder girdle** Arms	Eyes - Ears - Nose - Mouth Thyroid Heart Lungs Esophagus
T5-T9 Mid thorax	Local: Mid thoracic spine Ribs - Sternum **Shoulder girdle** Arms	Liver Gallbladder Stomach Adrenals Pancreas Spleen Duodenum
T10-L2 Thoraco-lumbar	Local: Thoraco-lumber spine Lower lumbar spine Sacrum Pelvis Legs	Small intestine Large intestine Kidneys Pelvic organs

Figure 1 - Segmental connections in the sympathetic nervous system. Red indicates the origin of the sympathetic neurons in the spinal cord and in the spinal cord foot reflex. Blue shows the origin of the parasympathetic nervous system (Brain stem + C1-C3 and S2-S4). Shoulder connections are highlighted. © 2011 Touchpoint Denmark

There are a few other techniques that are recommended. These include:

Linking

Linking is the primary technique of Precision Reflexology, developed by Prue Miskin. It involves holding two or three identified reflex points at the same time to work with subtle energy. The link is held, the practitioner pauses and 'listens' via their hands. Linking is initiated by stimulating the reflexes to be connected and feeling the energy between them.

This technique is about being intuitive to clients' energy and needs. The energy felt through the link should reflect the client: "An extremely energetic link (you will feel energy pulses, tingling and warmth) on a person who presents in a sluggish, lethargic manner could indicate an imbalance. However, on a lively person the same response would be regarded as normal" (Williamson J., Mark Allan publishing Ltd. p13). So to use linking, you simply place your thumbs and third fingers (positive energy) on the mentioned reflexes, close your eyes and think about what you can feel. If this is a new technique for you it can take a bit of practice, but it will become a valuable tool for you to use in any reflexology treatment.

Clients will respond in many different ways to a link; they may feel relaxed or warm through to feeling energised. They may feel sensations through their feet or through their whole body. Links can be used during a normal reflexology session to promote self-healing. Links should be held with thumbs and middle fingers as these contain positive receptors.

You can find some useful linking techniques on pages 151 and 152. All links that have been suggested in this book have been inspired by Jan Williamson's book, *A guide to Precision Reflexology* (2002).

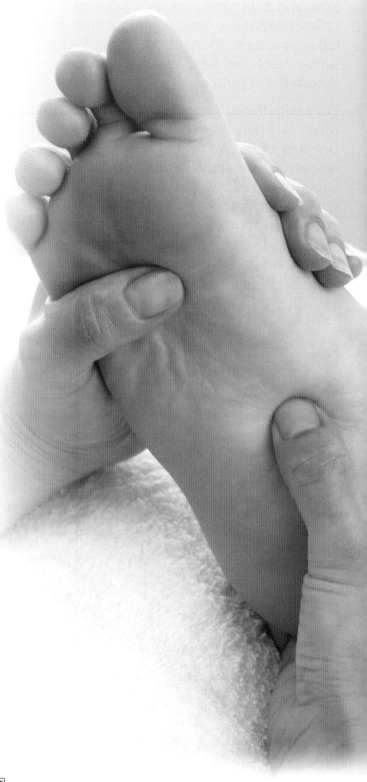

Williamson J. A guide to precision Reflexology. 2002. Mark Allan publishing Ltd. p12

Endocrine balance

This is an invaluable technique developed by Susanne Enzer designed for balancing hormones - and who wouldn't benefit from that?! It can be used for both men and women, and throughout the menstrual cycle.

Although the endocrine glands are found in different places around the body, they work as a unit, supporting and complementing each other. This endocrine balance therefore balances the entire system: body, mind and spirit

To access the physical energies, firm pressure is used, whilst light touch will access the emotions and feelings.

60

Method – this is a 4 step process

First identify the endocrine system reflex zones. Work both feet together with one hand on each foot.

1. Stimulate all the endocrine glands.

HYPOTHALAMUS – use the pads of the thumbs. Press firmly but gently into the reflex zones; bounce gently on the reflex	
PINEAL - thumb walk on the spot	
PITUITARY – Thumb walk on the spot	
THYROID - Thumb walk over the reflex zone. It easier to do this from lateral to medial	
THYMUS - use the 'thumb walking' area of the thumb. Thumb walk and tap the reflex zones	
PANCREAS - use the 'thumb walking' area of the thumb. Thumb walk the reflex zones – lateral to medial	
ADRENAL GLAND - use the pad of the thumb. Press gently into the reflex. Bounce gently on the reflexes until you feel a response	

OVARIES/TESTES – Place the thumb on the direct ovary/testes reflex and third finger on the indirect ovary/testes reflex. Make a pinch type movement of thumbs and fingers

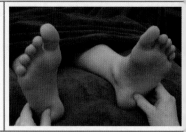

Now that all the endocrine glands are stimulated, they are ready for action. Connect them together to acknowledge that they are a unit. The connection movement is like a firm, stroking movement.

2. Connect the reflex zones of the endocrine system together by using a firm stroking movement from:

- Ovaries to adrenals.
- Adrenals to pancreas.
- Pancreas to thymus.
- Thymus to thyroid and parathyroid.
- Thyroid to pituitary.
- Pituitary to pineal.
- Pineal to hypothalamus.

3. Balance the reflex zones

- Repeat the connection but use a very light touch.
- Sense the energy under your fingers and set your intention to balance.
- If the energy feels the same, hold for several seconds and move onto the next zone in the sequence.
- If the energies do not feel the same, maintain the hold and the intention until you feel a balance or hold for up to 2 minutes.

4. Re-connect

If the energy does not balance in this time, complete the endocrine balance routine and return to the disordered gland. Consider using reflexology techniques to normalise it.

Method © Susanne Enzer: reproduced by kind permission

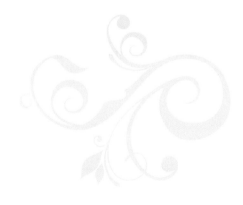

Concentrating on a reflex point or area

Below there are some recommended reflex points or areas that I have suggested you concentrate on or stimulate for different symptoms. This can mean you spend longer on the reflex, work it from different angles or revisit it several times during your treatment. You can try out different ways to see which you feel works best for you. To sedate a reflex, work gently and slowly and use your intention; think about your aim being to calm the area.

Reflex points and techniques for stress relief

Stress, over time, will affect all the body's systems so a full treatment is recommended to help reconnect the systems. The 'fight or flight' response starts with a combination of nerve impulses (sympathetic nervous system) and hormonal changes (directed by hypothalamus, pituitary and adrenal glands), so below are some reflexes and techniques.

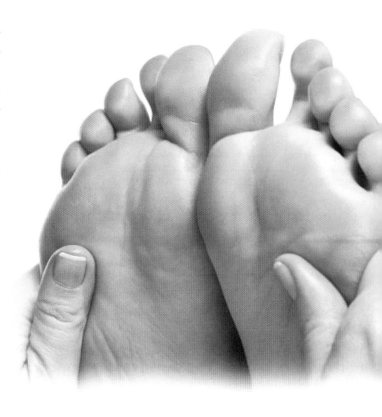

Reflex point	Reason
Adrenal glands	To calm the production of adrenalin
Head neck and shoulders	To relax tension
Solar plexus	To calm the individual
Spine – • sedate from T1 to L2 • Stimulate upper cervical spine and sacrum	To calm the sympathetic nervous system. To stimulate the parasympathetic nerves.
Endocrine balance (p61)	To support hormone balance
Linking – • Lumbar 5 to hip or • Pituitary, hypothalamus to adrenals	To relax the nervous system To help normalise the functioning of the Hypothalamic–pituitary–adrenal axis

Lumbar 5 to hip

Use one middle finger to locate lumbar 5 on the medial aspect of the foot and the other middle finger to hold the hip reflex.

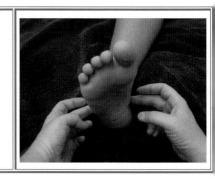

Pituitary and hypothalamus to adrenals

Use one thumb to rest on the pituitary reflex and the third finger to rest on the hypothalamus reflex. The other thumb rests on adrenal reflex.

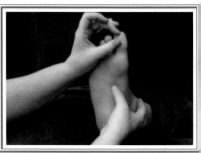

Reflexology for hormonal balance and supporting the reproductive system

Women

One of the first changes to ask your client to look for are changes in their hormonal balance. This may be changes in the length of their cycle, changes to their menstruation (e.g. if they were passing blood clots these should lessen), the heaviness of the bleed or they may notice emotional changes, hopefully with any PMS symptoms easing. Discuss these with your client after each period so they can begin to tune into their hormonal balance and begin to recognise any improvements.

Men and women

Much of the work on the endocrine system is again about getting the endocrine glands talking to each other. Detailed overleaf are some techniques that can be extremely useful in getting the endocrine glands working effectively and communicating with each other again.

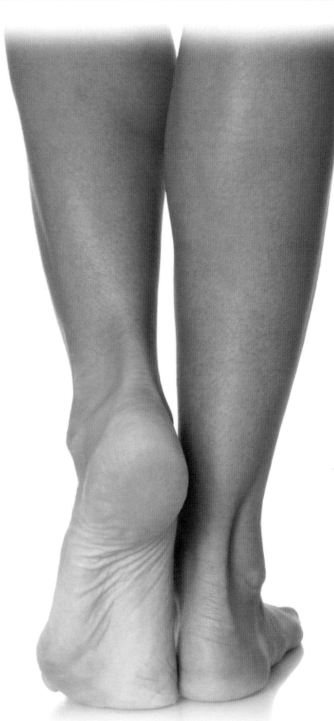

Toe Triangle

You will see that working the reflexes of the Toe Triangle is mentioned below; this term refers to pituitary, hypothalamus and pineal reflexes. Although the pineal reflex can be useful to work for circadian rhythms and sleep disturbance, it is often only the pituitary and hypothalamus that need to have more time spent working them. The reason I will refer to working the toe triangle is because I have trained many qualified reflexologists, and it soon came to my attention that the hypothalamus and pineal reflexes are often taught in different positions (i.e. just above pituitary is referred to as hypothalamus by some and pineal by others). If you look at different foot charts, you will also see these referred to in different positions. So rather than debating which is correct, it seemed sensible to include them as one sequence (Toe Triangle) to ensure all are covered.

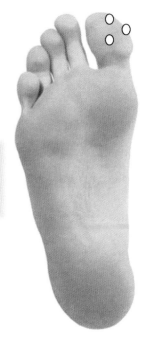

Toe Triangle:
- Pituitary
- Hypothalamus
- Pineal

Direct and indirect ovary/ testes reflex

The majority of reflexologists work the ovary/testes reflex on the lateral aspect of the foot in between the middle of the maleolus and the back of the heel. There is also another reflex called the direct ovary/ testes point located on the plantar aspect of the foot, just below the redness of the heel in zone 4. You can think of this as working the ovaries/testes from different aspects.

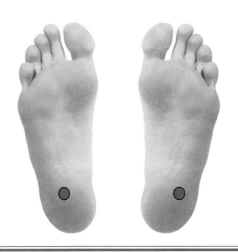

Direct ovary/testes reflexes

Pelvic Knuckling

The pelvic area is located at the back of the heel, on the lateral and medial aspects. Use your knuckles to work both sides at the same time. Use the flat surface of the knuckles for a gentle stimulation or the actual knuckle bones for a deeper working – this can be quite intense, so ensure your client is comfortable with this pressure. Working the pelvic area can help ease tension in the pelvic girdle and help communication between the ovaries/testes and uterus/prostate.

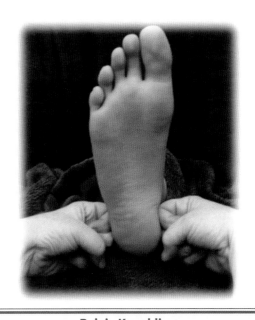

Pelvic Knuckling

Reproductive support sequence

This refers to a short sequence that can be repeated 4-6 times during a treatment:

- Toe Triangle
- Uterus/prostate
- Ovary/testes
- Direct ovary/testes
- Pelvic Knuckling

During your treatment, you can break regularly to carry out the reproductive stimulation sequence 4-6 times on each foot, spread throughout the treatment to encourage hormonal balance. When you work the toe triangle, follow this up with uterus/prostate reflex, ovary/testes reflex, direct ovary/testes point, and then knuckle the pelvic area to give a bit of 'caring' to the pelvic area.

Endocrine balance – see p61 and 62.

Reflexology sequence for hormonal balance.

You can use your full sequence but consider adding in the following techniques. This is largely about encouraging the endocrine system and nervous system to communicate and work effectively. Also remember that you will probably need to add in some of the reflexology recommended for stress.

Some useful techniques to consider

1. Spine – use 'open spine technique' and spinal twist - To clear central nervous system

Spinal Twist. Place both hands on top of the medial aspect of the foot. Lift the fore foot (lift the hand that is nearest the toes). Move both hands along the foot and repeat 2-3 times on each foot.	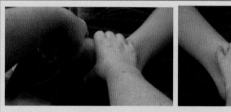 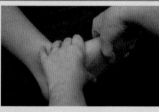
Open Spine Use your thumb to work along the spine, but your thumb moves perpendicular to the spine, thus working on the spinal nerves. Alternatively, use the side of your thumb to rub across the spine, place the side of your thumb on each vertebrae and rub across the spine - forwards and backwards (plantar to dorsal and then dorsal to plantar), so you are working across the spine rather than along it.	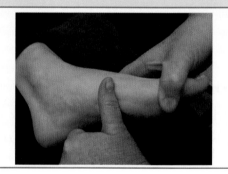

N.B. Spend plenty of time working the spine; do not rush it as the nervous system is essential for hormonal balance.

2. Reproductive support sequence - 4-6 times throughout your treatment

3. Toe Triangle, uterus/prostate, ovary/testes, direct ovary/testes, Pelvic Knuckling

4. Linking (see also p151 - 152) – there are several links which may be useful including:

Uterus, ovaries and adrenals/ Prostate, testes and adrenals The thumb and third finger of one hand holds the uterus and ovary (or prostate and testes) reflex points, whilst the thumb of the other hand holds the adrenal reflex.	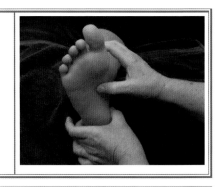
Uterus, ovaries and pituitary/ Prostate, testes and pituitary The thumb and third finger of one hand holds the uterus and ovary (or prostate and testes) reflex points, whilst the thumb of the other hand holds the pituitary reflex.	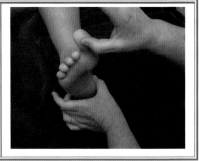

5. Endocrine balance – works well as a closing move

6. Other reflexes to consider – these may be useful on some clients:

Reflex point	Reason
Head and brain	To calm chemical imbalance.
Thyroid	The risk of infertility can be higher if the thyroid is not functioning adequately.
Pancreas	If a client with polycystic ovary syndrome has an issue with weight gain, stimulating the pancreas may help restore blood glucose levels.
Fallopian tubes / vas deferens	If there is a history of blockage or endometriosis, this may be helpful.
Large and small intestines	A healthy digestive system will help ensure the body is able to absorb nutrients and excrete waste.

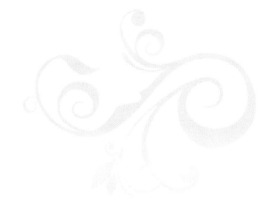

How to adapt your treatments throughout the menstrual cycle

When you are considering whether you will treat throughout the menstrual cycle, it is worth considering the two main phases; menstruation to ovulation and ovulation to conception/menstruation. If your client does not know when ovulation occurs, you can just divide the cycle in half and subtract 2 days (to be on the safe side) as a way to estimate the day of ovulation (i.e. in a 30 day cycle, half way would be day 15, subtract 2 days, so your estimated day of ovulation would be day 13). There are several thoughts on how you treat throughout the menstrual cycle; a few reflexologists choose not to treat at all after ovulation as the client could potentially be pregnant and as a reflexologist, you may not feel experienced enough to treat in the early stages of pregnancy. However, this approach has no evidence backing it and appears over cautious.

The two main approaches to deciding when and how to treat are discussed below. There is no evidence to say which the best approach is; our advice is to read both and reflect on which feels the correct approach for you:

1. *Alternating stimulation and relaxation*

This approach is based on using stimulating techniques (as described under reflexology for reproductive stimulation and hormone balance) from day 1 of the cycle until day of ovulation, and then a relaxing treatment (as described under reflexology for relaxation and stress relief) from day of ovulation until the next period begins or pregnancy is confirmed.

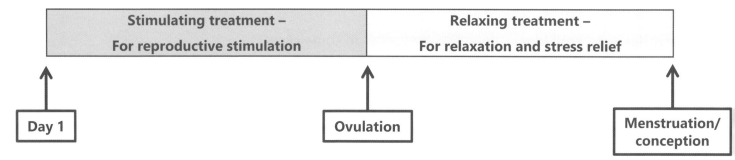

The stimulating treatment aims to optimise the functioning of the nervous and endocrine systems, reconnecting the systems to encourage the hormones to instruct the body correctly to build up a healthy endometrial lining in the uterus. Also, it is intended to initiate the maturing of an ovum and the release of the egg into the fallopian tubes ready for fertilization.

The relaxing treatment assumes that the major hormonal work has been done. By aiming to promote relaxation and stress relief at this time, the chance of fertilization will hopefully be optimised and then the body will be supported for implantation to take place.

2. *Stimulation until conception*

This approach recommends that the same treatment is used throughout the cycle until pregnancy is confirmed. The treatment should be a stimulating treatment, but should of course include some stress relief techniques.

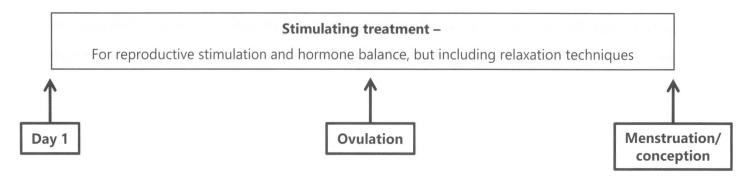

This approach recognises the usefulness of stimulating the nervous and endocrine systems before ovulation for the reasons stated above. However, after ovulation, this method is built around the fact that the body still has work to do. After ovulation, progesterone continues to rise and the endometrial lining continues to build so it is a healthy environment for a fertilized egg to implant into. It is also important that the fallopian tubes are functioning as well as they are able to, so the egg can be propelled along towards the uterus. Stimulation of the endocrine system may help to optimise functioning in this phase of the cycle.

The vast majority of clients will need some level of stress relief and will also benefit from stimulating the nervous and endocrine systems. This is where your intuition, knowledge and experience are needed to help you decide on how you will approach the treatment for that particular client.

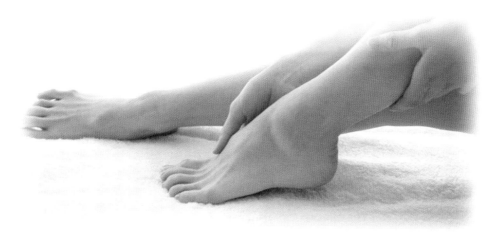

How to adapt your treatment for women during the IVF process

The processes involved in IVF have already been discussed, but where does reflexology fit in? I still hear reflexologists say "you can't treat during IVF" - but this is not the case. It may be that as an individual reflexologist you choose not to treat during IVF, and that is your choice. However, think of the stress levels that the couple is likely to be going through at this time; surely some relaxation and stress relief is just what they want? I suspect that the view that you should not treat has come from a 'fear' that reflexology may reverse the effects of the drugs involved; however, think of it in terms of:

IVF is bucket chemistry – reflexology is more subtle

This is a way of expressing that IVF involves metaphorical "buckets full of drugs" being emptied into the body, in far larger quantities than are actually required in normal circumstances. Reflexology works at a much more subtle level, so even if it causes the elimination of some of the drugs, there will still be plenty left. And think of the benefits to the client in terms of stress relief!

As a reflexologist, you need to make the initial decision as to whether you will treat during IVF or not. You must also think about how you would feel if the IVF was not successful - would you worry that the reflexology had made it fail? You need to remember that the chances of it succeeding are only about 1 in 3, and sometimes a pregnancy is simply not meant to be.

Assuming that you feel happy to go ahead, you do also need to discuss with the client that the reflexology will be aiming to aid relaxation and not trying to control hormone balance; they need to agree that they are happy to continue treatments whilst having IVF.

If either you or your client is unhappy about reflexology through IVF, make sure that you try to treat up until the day the client starts taking the drugs. There is one other window of time when she may really benefit from a reflexology session; encourage her to come back for 1 - 2 treatments in between egg retrieval and embryo transfer. This is a time when you can work on hormonal stimulation as there is only a short window for the body to start expelling all the drugs and for preparation of the uterus lining before the embryo is transferred. Also, stress levels are likely to be at an all time high at this time!

There are two time points when you might decide not to treat. The first is after the priming injection, which is given 36 hours prior to egg collection. If for whatever reason the client has no eggs to harvest it would be very easy to blame the reflexology, and this is a short time frame, so is easy to avoid. The second time point that you may decide not to treat is much longer and comes after embryo transfer; this is a time when the woman often metaphorically 'wraps herself in cotton wool'. It is the time after the embryo has been returned but before a positive pregnancy test or period. Remember, there is a one in three or less chance that the embryo transfer will result in pregnancy - it may be a good idea not to treat at this time so that if the embryo does not implant, it will not then be blamed on the reflexology or you. If the client absolutely wants treatment during this time and you are both comfortable to do so, then you can treat. But both of you must be happy, and you will need to make sure that if this is the case, the client signs to say that the reflexology was carried out at their request.

Below, the stages of IVF are listed with appropriate recommendations for reflexology.

Stage of the IVF cycle	To treat or not to treat?	Approach
Before IVF begins	Yes	Hormonal stimulation and stress relief
During downregulation	Yes, if you and your client are happy	Stress relief
During upregulation	Yes, if you and your client are happy	Stress relief
After priming injection (for maturation of the eggs)	No	This is an easily avoided 36 hour time slot and should the eggs be released accidentally during this phase it could be blamed on reflexology
After egg retrieval	Yes	Hormonal stimulation, detoxification and stress relief
After embryo transfer	WITH CAUTION – only if client and reflexologist are happy to do so	Wait until pregnancy is confirmed or not.

How often should I treat the client who wishes to conceive?

On the first consultation, explain to your client that you would like them to commit to six months of reflexology, and ideally see both partners. In an ideal world, it would be beneficial for clients to have weekly treatments for 6 weeks, then treatments every 2 weeks for a couple of months and then they can move onto monthly treatments – obviously this is a rough guide and you will need to assess progress as you go along.

However, many people cannot commit to that frequency of treatments, often due to financial and/or time constraints. You need to discuss, as you would with any client, what is an acceptable treatment plan for them. If they can only see you monthly, it is generally believed that it is best to see them before ovulation (or estimated ovulation).

Remember that these clients may often have high levels of stress, anxiety and/or depression, so they may need time to talk about this. However, it is also essential that they do have time to close their eyes during the treatment to ground themselves, remember what being relaxed feels like and maybe to spend some time visualising themselves either pregnant or holding their baby to help them believe they can conceive.

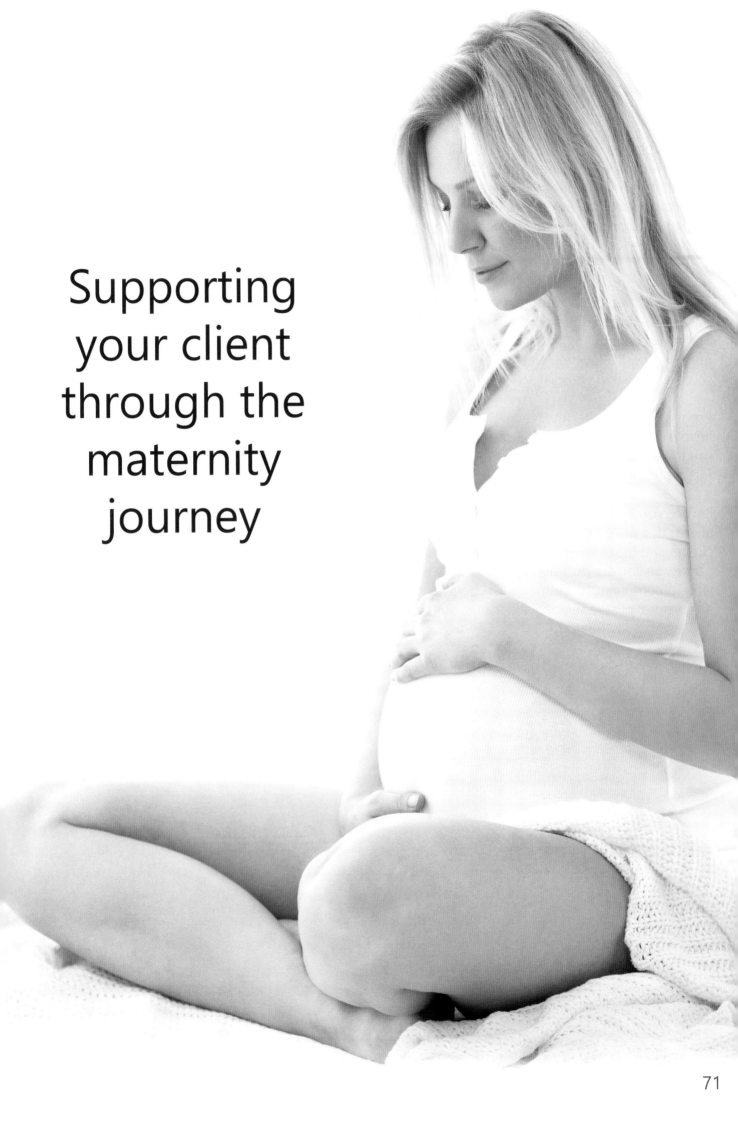

Supporting your client through the maternity journey

Introduction to *reflexology through the maternity journey*

Being able to support women with reflexology through their pregnancy and beyond is a wonderful experience and one that we should feel honoured to be a part of. Reflexology during pregnancy aims to optimise the health of the pregnant woman and it is important that you do not treat pregnancy as an illness. Concentrate on treating any conditions that arise during pregnancy and offer support and advice accordingly. As a reflexologist you may give reflexology and general lifestyle advice, but you must not at any time give medical or obstetric guidance; you must ensure that a client with problems is in the care of the appropriate clinical practitioners.

This guide has been designed to give you information to help you treat and support pregnant and post natal women. It is important that you understand the basic physiology of foetal development and the maternal changes that happen throughout the pregnancy – all of this information will be covered in this guide and will allow you to talk knowledgeably to the mother. You will be able to reassure her that what she is experiencing is normal or suggest she talks to her midwife if you are concerned about her symptoms.

Pregnancy and maternity is a huge subject area; this guide will only focus on the more common issues that arise in pregnancy and is not a substitute for additional training; if you would like to progress in treating pregnant clients and be able to state that you are experienced in doing so, you need to gain experience and further training. **Appendix 1** shows a diagram that has been devised to show the route you need to take.

Before you continue to read on, **it is essential that you read and digest the maternity information sheet;** this will give you all the information you need to know about when it is not safe to treat maternity clients and times when you need to treat with caution. This information must be adhered to at all times, otherwise you are putting yourself and your client at potential risk and your insurance would not be valid were a complaint to be made. Do be aware that this book is for information and guidance only; if you are unsure, please seek advice from a suitably qualified expert.

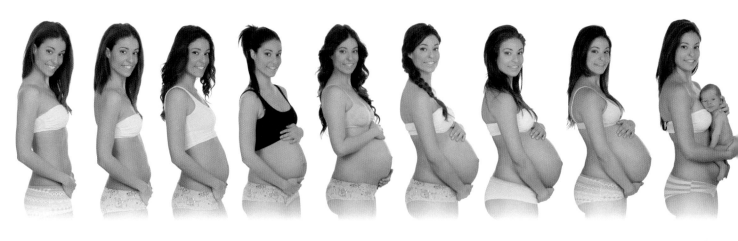

Treating pregnant women:
The AoR information sheet

Can I treat in the first trimester of pregnancy?

There are a number of issues that need to be examined when answering this. While there are risks throughout pregnancy, there is a higher likelihood of miscarriage in the first three months/13 weeks of pregnancy.

Therefore, if you provide reflexology for someone during this period, there is statistically a greater chance that they will miscarry than if they were treated later on in the pregnancy. This is nature's quality control in action. There is no evidence to show that reflexology can bring on a miscarriage. Indeed, some reflexologists claim that reflexology can be used effectively in situations where there has been a history of miscarriage, though once again, there is no research evidence to back this up. If, as is supposed, reflexology works by helping the body to function correctly, then should a miscarriage occur at some point during a course of reflexology treatments, the conclusion could be drawn that this is the body's natural response to a problem with the pregnancy.

Once again though, there is no scientific evidence to demonstrate that reflexology does work in this way. Both the client and therapist need to understand and accept this concept before treatment can begin.

Pregnancy is an extremely emotive area, and it is recommended that only reflexologists with at least one year's experience should consider treating clients who are under 13 weeks pregnant. To help with developing the skills and judgements required for practising safely in this area, members are recommended to attend one of the growing number of Continuing Professional Development (CPD) workshops or courses covering pregnancy and childbirth. If you are going to embark on further training, please make sure that the reflexologist who is delivering the course is suitably qualified and experienced. Ideally, these courses will be offered by reflexologists with medical training, who have at least five years' reflexology experience and three years' experience in treating pregnant clients. Your course should also contain a case study element. You should also try to find a workshop leader who will give you backup support following the course.

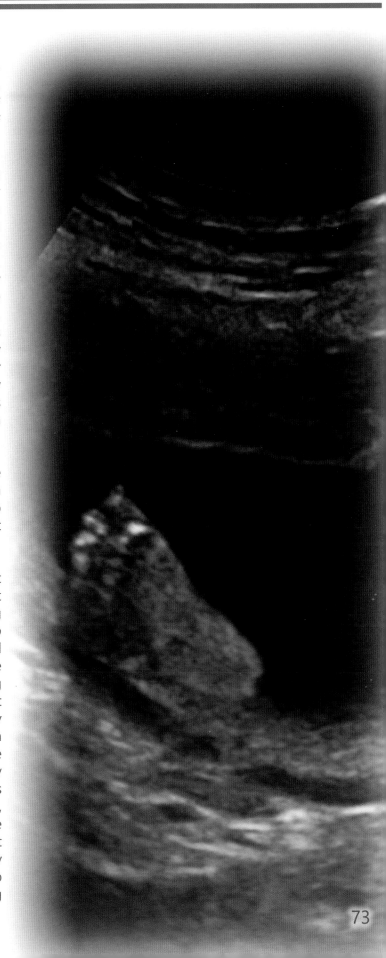

When is treatment contraindicated?

The following situations are contraindicated and must not be treated:

- DVT: this is a standard contraindication.

- Pre-eclampsia: fluid retention, high blood pressure and protein in the urine, this will be diagnosed by the midwife or doctor.

- Pre-term labour (less than 37 weeks pregnant): as it is not counted as normal; your client should contact her midwife/GP or hospital.

- Placenta Previa (low lying afterbirth) if Grade II, III, or IV and 32 weeks or more: it can be fatal to both mother and baby if the placenta comes off the uterine wall as it grows and stretches, causing severe bleeding.

- Polyhydramnios (excessive liquor around the foetus which can be linked to congenital abnormalties and risk the cord prolapsing and becoming compressed): if it is mild the client can be treated with midwife/doctor agreement. If it is severe this can be life threatening and the mother risks losing the baby should membranes rupture, as the presenting part is not engaged. The client is likely to be in hospital and should only be treated with Consultant approval.

- Oligohydramnios (the lack of fluid around the baby): if it is mild the client can be treated with midwife/doctor agreement. If it is severe this can be linked to kidney problems in the baby, and puts the baby at risk as there is not enough cushioning to protect it. The client is likely to be in hospital and should only be treated with Consultant approval.

- Placental abruption: when the placenta separates from the wall of the uterus.

Other situations

Both reflexologist and client must be completely happy with the treatment going ahead, and if there is any doubt in either's mind, then treatment is contraindicated

To establish whether the client is happy to receive reflexology, they must be in receipt of all the information, have had an opportunity to discuss the issue with you and have any questions answered to their satisfaction. Only then can the client make an informed choice

Dos and don'ts

- Do focus on the client's health.

- Do take extra care to ensure client comfort.

- Do allow extra time between ending the session and the client standing up.

- Do research and understand your subject.

- Do attend a CPD workshop/course on pregnancy.

- Don't exceed your training and experience.

- Don't treat pregnancy as an illness.

- Don't lie your client flat in the third trimester during treatment, and do be aware of the risk of supine hypotension.

- Don't have the room too warm.

- Be aware of smells in the treatment room – some pregnant women have a very sensitive sense of smell!

To establish whether you, as the reflexologist, are happy to provide reflexology, you must have provided all the information to the client, discussed their circumstances and answered all their questions to both their and your satisfaction.

You must also be in the position where, if the client were to miscarry following a reflexology session, you would be able to deal with the client appropriately, and be able to cope emotionally yourself with the inevitable upset and self-questioning that will follow.

History of unstable pregnancies

In the past this has always been an area where contra-indication is absolute. However, there is some anecdotal evidence suggesting that there may be benefits to treating someone who has a history of miscarriage or who has a medical diagnosis of unstable pregnancy during the first three months of pregnancy. Such is the level of caution required in these circumstances that it is recommended that only

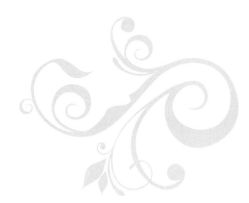

reflexologists with a depth of knowledge, understanding and experience in this area should even contemplate taking on clients in this category. To add to this, it is recommended that your client should contact their doctor regarding receiving reflexology. Following this, all the considerations concerning contraindications and cautions apply, in particular the ability of the reflexologist to cope with any eventuality.

'Are there any reflex points that I should avoid?'

The only point thought to possibly induce miscarriage in acupuncture is Spleen 6. This is on the medial side of the ankle, about two-and-a-half finger widths up from the medial malleolus. As this is not a universally taught reflex point that is part of a regular reflexology session, there should be no reason to work on this reflex.

Some schools teach that the ovaries, uterus, pituitary and thyroid should be avoided at all times throughout pregnancy. Current information suggests that there is no reason to avoid these reflexes, but neither is it recommended that you should specifically work into these areas. Nevertheless, avoidance of these points for the first 36 weeks of pregnancy provides some extra points to concentrate on during the last four weeks.

Treatment during pregnancy is generally focused on helping the client to have a healthy and trouble-free pregnancy. This involves a fairly standard approach to the treatment session, not focusing on any reflexes in particular, other than those which will help the client to manage their health successfully whilst pregnant.

'Can I use reflexology to induce labour?'

Once again, there is some anecdotal evidence to suggest that reflexology can help to bring on labour, providing both mother and baby are ready. It is always recommended that those clients who wish to use reflexology for this purpose begin their reflexology sessions at least six weeks prior to their predicted term date i.e. before they are 34 weeks pregnant. It is useful to use a term such as 'preparation for labour' rather than inducing as this helps manage expectations.

It is recommended that you do not use labour-inducing techniques unless the client has received at least two reflexology sessions in the two or three weeks prior to term and they are past their due date. If you were to carry out a deep stimulating treatment for a first treatment this could potentially increase the risk of a healing reaction and you don't want them go into labour already feeling sick or with a headache.

It is also worth reassuring clients that sometimes a relaxing treatment is all that is needed, as if the body is in state of fight or flight; if they feel worried about the labour, this can be enough to inhibit the onset of labour as the body is saying it needs to escape from danger first. Therefore, the first two treatments should concentrate on relaxation and then you can start to include some preparation for labour techniques.

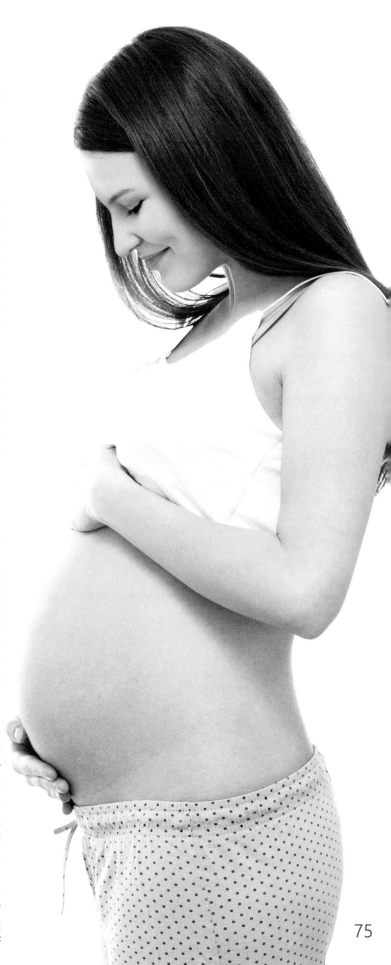

Areas of caution

The following situations need to be diagnosed and, if appropriate, treated by a midwife or doctor before you commence reflexology. You need to be very honest with yourself about how experienced you are as a reflexologist in having encountered a wide variety of situations and disorders.

- Multiple Pregnancies (twins, triplets, etc.).

- Vaginal Discharge can be normal increased physiological discharge, mucous from labour, blood from labour or haemorrhage, liquor from ruptured membranes.

- Uterine Pain can be the onset of labour, kidney infection, scar pain from a previous caesarean section, bleeding from the placenta.

- Epilepsy, as it can get worse during pregnancy and will need careful monitoring.

- Diabetes, as this too can get worse during pregnancy and needs monitoring carefully.

- Any other health problems which might affect your client adversely during her pregnancy – e.g. heart, kidney or liver disorders.

- If at any time you don't feel happy or confident, or if any changes occur then the client must be advised to contact their doctor.

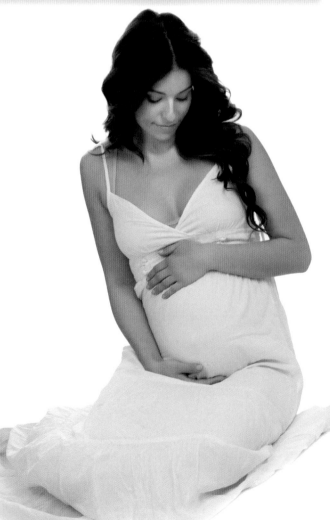

Miscarriage

A miscarriage refers to the loss of a pregnancy before 23 weeks. It is estimated that the rate of miscarriage is somewhere between 15-20%, and approximately 1% have recurrent miscarriages (three or more consecutive miscarriages), these women will usually be offered tests to look for causes.

There are probably many reasons why a miscarriage may happen, but reassure your client that the majority aren't caused by anything the mother has done, but rather are caused by abnormal chromosomes in the baby. There are some lifestyle factors that increase the risk e.g. obesity, smoking, alcohol, and the risk of miscarriage increases after the age of 35, but the cause often remains unknown.

After a miscarriage a study has shown that 1 in 5 women express high levels of anxiety and up to a third are diagnosed with depression(1). So with clients be aware these can be significant issues and remember they will also be grieving for the loss of their unborn baby.
For more information visit:

www.tommys.org

www.nhs.uk/Conditions/Miscarriage/Pages/Causes.aspx

References

(1) Rai R, Regan L, Recurrent miscarriage. Lancet 2006; 368(9535): 601-11

Conclusion

Pregnancy is a very difficult, emotive and individual area, which necessitates a high degree of caution, and for which there is no substitute for training and experience. These AoR guidelines have been put together in consultation with very experienced and highly qualified reflexologists and members of the medical profession.

Should you be interested in developing these techniques further, it is suggested that you attend a pregnancy and childbirth workshop run by a suitably qualified and experienced tutor.

Out of necessity, some areas are generalised in this book and there may be a number of clients who do not fit neatly into the guidelines. If you are concerned whether your training and experience allows you to practise on a particular client, please contact the AoR Helpline on 01823 351010 to discuss the case in more detail.

An introduction to *the three trimesters of pregnancy*

Pregnancy is generally said to last 40 weeks. The due date is calculated from the first day of the last normal menstrual cycle; this is based on Naegele's rule, which was developed in the early 19th century. As fertilization takes place approximately 2 weeks after the start of the last menstrual cycle, the woman is technically not pregnant for the first 2 weeks of the 40 week period.

> **Pregnancy is also often talked about in terms of three trimesters; these are arbitrary landmarks during the pregnancy:**
>
> The first trimester (1-13 weeks): characterised by huge hormonal changes, implantation of the embryo into the uterine wall and development of the foetus.
>
> The second trimester (14-27 weeks): discomforts of first trimester have passed and most women begin to feel incredibly well. The baby begins to grow.
>
> The third trimester (28-40 weeks): the baby continues to mature and grow, and this increase in size may begin to cause strain on the mother's body.

This guide will look at each trimester, labour and the post-natal period in terms of changes that are occurring, advice that can be given and how to adapt your reflexology for each stage.

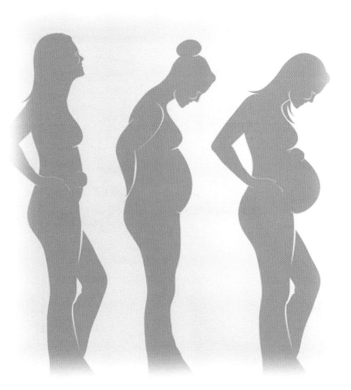

Hormones in Maternity

Pregnancy is largely governed by hormones; production of existing hormones is raised and new hormones are made. It is important that you have a basic understanding of the roles that different hormones have in pregnancy and where they are produced. The main players are:

- **Human Chorionic Gonadotrophin (hCG):** this is released by the developing placenta and triggers other hormones that are required to maintain a pregnancy. This is the hormone that is tested for in pregnancy tests and is thought to be a cause of morning sickness.

- **Progesterone:** Levels of progesterone are significantly higher in a pregnant woman. This hormone is produced primarily by the ovaries and later by the placenta.

Progesterone has many roles; it:

➢ prevents the uterus from contracting during pregnancy.

➢ maintains the placenta, strengthens the pelvic walls and relaxes ligaments and muscles in preparation for labour.

➢ prepares the breasts for milk production by developing the duct system in the breasts; this can cause tenderness.

The relaxant effect on muscles and ligaments can also cause bowels to become sluggish, veins to dilate (increasing the chance of varicose veins and haemorrhoids), and relaxes the sphincter between the oesophagus and stomach, causing heartburn in some women.

Oestrogen levels are also higher during pregnancy, which helps to build the uterus lining ready for implantation and increases blood volume ready for the extra demands on the woman's body. This also means that nosebleeds and bleeding gums are more common, together with increased redness and flushing of the skin.

Other hormones involved in pregnancy are;

- **Human Chorionic Somatomammotropin (HCS),** which is regulated by oestrogen and is produced by the placenta.

  It aids development of the foetus, helps breasts develop and allows fat to be converted into energy.

- **Thyroxine,** which is produced in the thyroid gland and is needed for the development of the central nervous system of the foetus. It also interacts with growth hormones to allow the foetus to grow and process proteins and carbohydrates.

- **Calcitonin,** which is also produced in the thyroid gland and acts to reduce blood calcium levels to protect bone strength during pregnancy.

- **Relaxin,** which is produced by the corpus luteum (on the ovary where the egg has been released) and later by the placenta. It helps the cervix, pelvic muscles, ligaments and joints to relax in preparation for labour.

- **Insulin,** which is produced by the pancreas and helps the foetus to store food and regulate glucose levels.

- **Oxytocin,** which is produced by the pituitary gland, and is important during labour and the post-natal period. It is released in large amounts once the cervix begins to stretch during labour; it then causes the uterus to contract, aiding birth. After the birth, oxytocin is released if the nipples are stimulated during breastfeeding and causes the breast milk to flow.

- **Erythropoietin,** which is produced by the kidneys to increase the total mass of red blood cells to cope with the increased demand for oxygen.

- **Cortisol,** which is produced by the adrenal glands; levels increase between weeks 30-32 to help the lungs of the foetus to mature.

- **Prolactin,** which is produced primarily in the pituitary gland, but also in the breasts and uterine lining. Increased levels during pregnancy cause enlargement of the breasts ready for milk production and then stimulate lactation (milk production) after the birth.

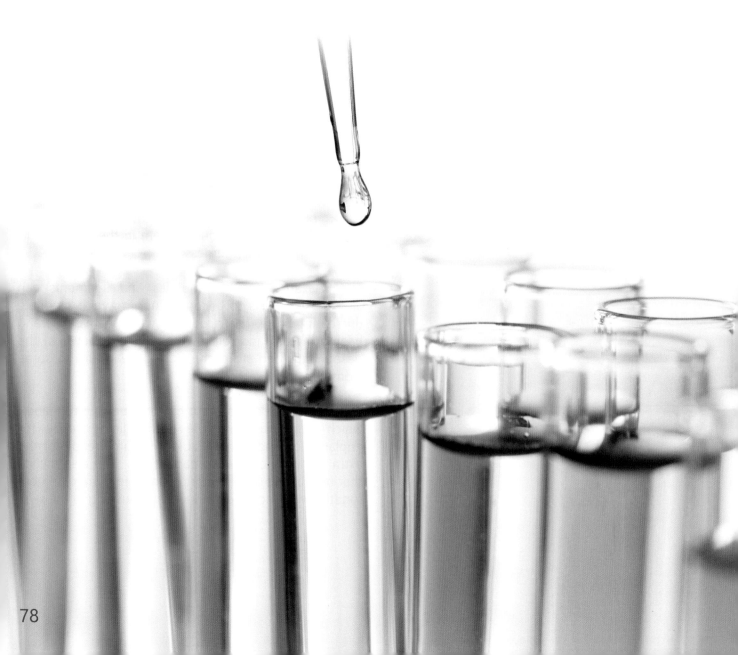

First trimester- Weeks 1-13

The first 13 weeks of pregnancy are generally referred to as the first trimester and this is a time of rapid development, governed by hormones. After fertilization, the zygote (fertilized egg cell or cells) will begin to multiply rapidly, and this solid bundle of cells (now called a morula) continues to travel along the fallopian tubes towards the uterus, which takes approximately 7 days. When the morula reaches the uterus it will contain approximately 64 cells; a few of these will develop into the embryo - the rest will form the placenta and the membranes that surround the baby. In this time, the morula changes from being a solid ball of cells into a ball of cells containing fluid, and at this stage is referred to as a blastocyst. Once the blastocyst has reached the uterus, it will endeavour to implant into the uterine wall. At this time progesterone levels are at their highest, stimulating the blood supply to the endometrium (lining of the uterus) to prepare the uterus for implantation of the blastocyst.

Implantation happens between day 6 and day 12 following fertilization; the outer layer of the blastocyst (trophoblastic cells) develops sponge like projections which are able to burrow into the uterine wall. These cells grow into chorionic villi which will later develop into the placenta.

After implantation, the blastocyst releases enzymes that break down the endometrium to allow the blastocyst to receive nourishment from the blood supply of the uterine lining. Occasionally, there are not enough nutrients supplied to the blastocyst and this results in a miscarriage, which manifests as a late, heavy period.

After implantation, the rapidly developing new life is referred to as an embryo. The embryo is able to produce its own progesterone to allow the endometrium to develop further, in order to continue providing the nourishment required. At this stage, the internal organs of the embryo begin to develop.

By 8 weeks, all the major organs have formed in the embryo and it is now referred to as a foetus. By the end of the first trimester the foetus is recognizably human with arms, legs, fingers, toes and even nails.

When considering a pregnancy, as discussed in the first chapter, the 'due date' is calculated from the last menstrual cycle, but fertilization does not occur until about 2 weeks later. This means that the woman is not actually pregnant for the first 2 weeks of the notional 40 week pregnancy.

Human Embryonic and Foetal Development

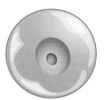 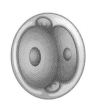 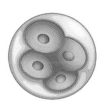 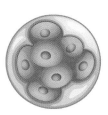 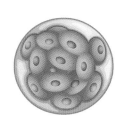 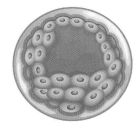

Fertilized egg   2-cell stage   4-cell stage   8-cell stage   16-cell stage   Blastocyst

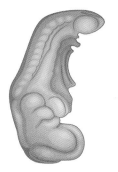 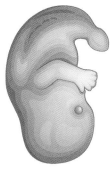

Foetus - 4 weeks   Foetus - 10 weeks

Terminology:

Time from fertilization	Week of pregnancy	Term used	Development
Day 1	3	Zygote - fertilized egg cell	Zygote rapidly divides and moves towards the uterus.
Day 4	3	Morula	Solid bundle of cells.
Day 6-7	3	Blastocyst Cell cluster	A fluid filled ball of cells. Cells continue to divide into 3 layers which will perform different functions.
Up to week 8	3-10	Embryo	The blastocyst implants into the uterine wall. Outer cells burrow deeply into the endometrium to form the placenta. Within the blastocyst, an embryonic disc forms to provide a fluid-filled sac (amniotic cavity) in which the embryo can grow.
Week 8	10	Foetus	Cells begin to differentiate into the various body systems. After 8 weeks, all the major body organs have now developed and the embryo becomes known as a foetus for the remaining term of the pregnancy.

Foetal development

After the embryo has implanted into the uterine wall, the placenta develops to become the organ that connects the developing foetus to the uterine wall. This provides nutrients to the foetus, allowing waste products to be eliminated and gas exchange to take place from the mother's blood supply.

The placenta forms from uterine cells and the cells from the outer layer of the embryo. An umbilical cord grows, connecting the foetus to the placenta. With the provision of nutrients and oxygen and efficient removal of waste products, the tremendous growth starts and changes can really begin. The foetus develops over the following 32 weeks inside the amniotic sac, which provides protection from knocks and bumps.

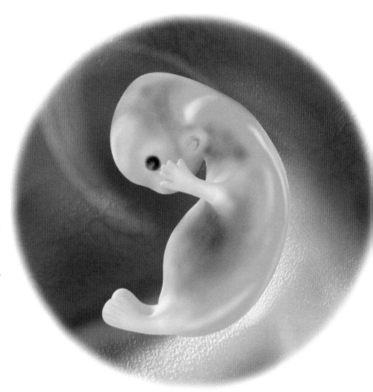

Week of pregnancy	Development
3	Fertilization occurs.
3-4	Implantation; pregnancy tests can detect the pregnancy.
5	The embryo starts to develop skin and all body organs and systems begin to develop.
6	The embryo begins to develop arms, legs and basic facial features.
7	The brain, face, arms and legs have developed fully.
8	The embryo starts to move, although it will not be felt by the mother until it is larger.
9-12	The toes, neck and genitals develop.

By the end of the first trimester the foetus will be approximately 7.5cm and will weigh approximately 45g (1).

The first trimester from the woman's perspective

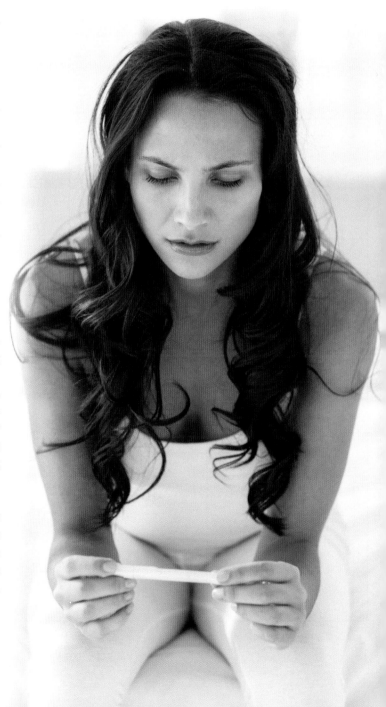

The first trimester of pregnancy can be a rollercoaster for some pregnant women; there is often excitement, followed by tears and concerns. Physically, there may be nausea, tiredness and tender breasts. Other women may just breeze through these first 3 months, others may struggle to even get out of bed – each woman's experience will be different, so it is vital that you listen to each client's story and appreciate that how they are feeling will change from day to day, or indeed from minute to minute.

Confirming the pregnancy

Some women just know instinctively that they are pregnant, where others may have no inclination at all. Some of the more common symptoms (these will discussed later in detail) are morning sickness, changes in taste and smell, tiredness and breast tenderness. The clearest indication is missing a period. Two weeks after fertilization, the placenta is starting to form and begins to produce the hormone human chorionic gonadatrophin (hCG).

Home pregnancy tests can confirm pregnancy at this stage by detecting hCG in urine. These are very accurate and will generally be accepted as confirmation of pregnancy. If the urine test is inconclusive, a GP may do a blood test to confirm pregnancy.

References

(1) Human Body, DK pg. 262.

Second trimester - Weeks 14-27

The second trimester of pregnancy is often the most enjoyable, as many of the symptoms experienced in the first trimester (e.g. morning sickness) begin to disappear; this is the stage when women are often referred to as 'blooming'. This also tends to be the least stressful time in the pregnancy; worries of miscarriage begin to ease and the anxiety of giving birth is still a long way off. Another reassurance is that along with the growing abdomen, this is when the first movements of the foetus are usually felt and this helps the pregnancy to feel more real. Although the foetus has been constantly moving around in the womb, it is not until the second trimester that the foetus is large enough for the movements to be felt. The first movements are usually felt around weeks 18-20, although sometimes earlier if it is not a first pregnancy.

Foetal development

By the end of the first trimester, the foetus is fully formed. As the second trimester starts, the growth of the foetus begins to speed up and internal organs begin to mature.

Week	Approximate size of foetus	Foetal developments
14	8-9 cm	• Nervous system begins to function • Foetus begins to bend and flex joints • Hair begins to appear on the head • Placenta will soon be developed enough to take over the production of hormones • Red blood cells are forming in the spleen
15	10 cm	• Bones begin to develop • Ribs, blood vessels and retinas are visible • Skin becomes covered with fine hairs to help regulate body temperature • Auditory system begins to develop
16	11 cm	• Bones begin to ossify (become harder) • Foetus' sex organs have developed and the gender of the baby can be identified (from an ultrasound scan)
17	11-12 cm	• Fat begins to be laid down under the skin • Foetus can now hear sounds from outside the womb • Practice breathing movements are taking place
18	12-14 cm	• Foetus is becoming increasingly active, twisting, turning, punching and kicking • Alveoli develop in the lungs
19	13-15 cm	• Foetus develops a waterproof covering called vernix caseosa to protect it from the amniotic fluid • Myelin sheaths begins to form around the foetus' nerve cells • Gastric juices are produced • Amniotic fluid is absorbed, passed to kidneys to be filtered and then excreted.

Week	Approximate size of foetus	Foetal developments
20	14-16 cm	• Half way! • Rapid growth continues • Sensory organs develop – taste, hearing, sight and smell
21	16-17 cm	• Brain nerve endings are developed enough that the foetus can sense touch and may begin thumb sucking and stroking
22	19cm	• Brain begins to grow rapidly • Sweat glands are formed in the skin
23	20 cm	• Foetus can now distinguish different voices; once the baby is born, he/she will be able to recognise voices first heard in the womb. The mother and father should both be encouraged to talk to their baby from this time.
24	21 cm	• White blood cells start to be produced
25	22 cm	• Teeth begin to form in the gums • Nerves around lips develop ready for feeding
26	23 cm	• Spine becomes stronger and more supple • Eyes are completely formed
27	24 cm	• Fat is laid down under the skin • Lungs continue to grow and develop • Eyelids can now open

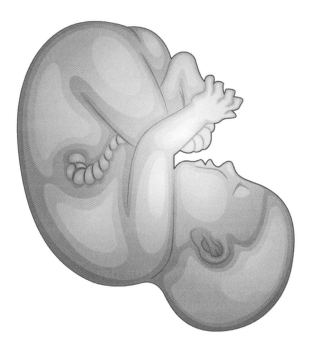

Foetus - 20 weeks

Changes in the mother's body

As hormonal changes begin to level out in the second trimester, women tend to feel more relaxed and are less prone to mood swings. Although this tends to be the most enjoyable trimester for the woman, there are still plenty of changes that occur in her body. She will now be having regular ante-natal checks to monitor the heartbeat and growth of the foetus.

Growth of the uterus

As the foetus grows, so does the mother's womb; from week 15 onwards, the mother will need to consider wearing maternity clothes to prevent constriction of the foetus. From about 17 weeks, the mother will be able to sense a fluttering feeling in her womb as the baby is moving around. The normal weight gain should be around 1.5 – 2kg per month.

Third trimester - Weeks 28-40

The third trimester is predominantly a time of rapid growth for the foetus, which may gain up to 28g per day. The foetus lays down fat to help preserve heat and his/her muscle tone is getting better. The foetus is often on the move and these movements can become quite strong and uncomfortable. Whilst a woman is receiving reflexology, punches and kicks can often be seen through her clothing, particularly whilst you are working around the uterus and pelvic area.

Some women find that they feel great during this last 3 months, whilst others may struggle with symptoms such as back ache, exhaustion, constipation, heartburn, breathlessness, etc.

As the birth becomes more imminent, anxiety about the birth is common and this can feel overwhelming at times. Some women may also get ante-natal depression possibly as a result of their anxiety over the birth, tiredness and generally being fed up with being pregnant. It is important to note that those women who become depressed prior to the birth are at higher risk of post-natal depression.

Foetal development

As stated above, the main development in the third stage is growth and weight gain; also, the lungs are still immature. It is possible for a baby to be born and survive now, but they may need assistance to breathe.

Week	Approximate size of foetus	Foetal developments
28	25cm	• For boys, the testes begin to descend into the scrotum • Foetus is laying down fat and plumping out many of the wrinkles on his/her skin
29	26cm	• Foetus is unable to turn as freely now, but will still be kicking and punching • Bones are fully developed but still soft • Rapid brain growth
30	27cm	• Brain, muscles and lungs continue to mature • Skeleton is hardening • Bone marrow is now able to produce red blood cells • Foetus usually moves to the head down position from this time. Kicks will be under the ribcage when this happens
31	28cm	• Eyes are opening and closing, pupils start to dilate, and eye colour will begin to appear – although this will change during the first 6 months after birth • Foetus can now control body temperature
32	29cm	• All five senses are working • Practice breathing movements continue to help the development of the lungs • The foetus sleeps for up to 90% of the day
33	30cm	• Kicking and hitting become less frequent now as there is little space, although the mother will still feel the baby shifting around

Week	Approximate size of foetus	Foetal developments
34	31cm	• Immune system is developing • Digestive system is almost complete
35	32cm	• By now, 99% of babies would survive being born • Lungs are close to being mature
36	33cm	• The majority will now be head down, but 3-4% will present in the breech position (bottom or legs facing the cervix). • The head may begin to move down into the pelvic cavity and pressure will be increased on the pelvic floor • Movements are less frequent but are stronger
37	34cm	• Foetus is now considered full term!! All organs should be ready to function on their own • If the foetus is in the breech presentation, a doctor may attempt to manually turn the baby by external manipulation (external cephalic version)
38	35cm	• Foetus has developed a strong grasp • Waste material (meconium) is building up in the intestines which will usually be passed after birth. Any meconium (brown or black tarry substance) passed in the liquor when the membranes rupture requires urgent assessment, as this can indicate foetal distress or post maturity • Placenta starts to become less efficient
39-42	36-37cm	• A waiting game!! It is generally considered safe to go one or two weeks over the due date. The midwife will be keeping a very close eye on things now to ensure the mum and baby are well and happy.

Changes in the mother's body

As the mother enters her last three months of pregnancy, many find it physically demanding as the growth of the foetus begins to push on many of the mother's organs. It is also a time when anxieties about the birth can begin to mount. Generally, women may now be having fortnightly ante-natal checks, increasing to once a week after week 36 (this timing may vary slightly with different NHS Trusts). These checks are an excellent time for the woman to discuss any concerns with a health care professional.

Continued breast growth.

By now, there might be an additional kilogram of breast tissue. As delivery approaches, the nipples could start leaking colostrum (the yellowish fluid that will nourish the baby during the first few days of life).

Weight gain

By the due date, women should expect to weigh about 11 to 16 kilograms more than they did before pregnancy. The baby accounts for some of the weight gain, but so do the placenta, amniotic fluid, larger breasts, larger uterus, extra fat stores, and increased blood and fluid volume.

Labour

Every woman's experience of labour is unique; even a woman who has several children will have a different experience each time. And why is it that women who have had a bad birthing experience seem to be the only ones who share their stories? I certainly know plenty of women who have managed labour extremely well. So if a client comes in and shares with you horror stories that she has heard, reassure her that the majority of women cope fine.

There is no way to predict what sort of labour any woman will have, but remember to tell your clients that two recent studies have shown that reflexology in pregnancy significantly reduced pain during labour (1), reduced the length of the first stage of labour (1) and improved quality of sleep in post-natal women (2).

(1) VALIANI M ET AL (2010) Reviewing the effect of Reflexology on pain and outcomes of the labour of primiparous women. Iranian Journal of Nursing and Midwifery Research. 15(Dec) p302-310

(2) LI C-Y ET AL (2011) Randomised controlled trial of the effectiveness of using foot reflexology to improve quality of sleep amongst post partum women. Midwifery. 27. p181-186

Labour is described as having three stages:

- Stage 1: opening and thinning of the cervix
- Stage 2: birth of the baby
- Stage 3: delivery of the placenta

The exact cause of the onset of labour remains a bit of a mystery. The one thing that is for sure is that the woman will know when she has well and truly started the first stage. Labour is defined as starting when contractions become regular, have a rhythmic pattern, last longer and start to dilate the cervix.

However there are changes that will occur as the birth approaches, but do not actually indicate that labour is about to start; labour could still be days or weeks away.

These include:

- Head becomes engaged: the lower part of the uterus softens and expands, and the head descends lower into the pelvis (the term used is engaged). For first pregnancies, this usually happens two to four weeks before labour starts, but with subsequent pregnancies it may only happen when labour begins. When the foetus drops down into the pelvis, this is the time when breathing and heartburn may ease. However, lower pelvic pressure can then cause increased back ache, oedema in feet, ankles and legs, and even more frequent urination.

- Vaginal discharge: This may increase as the cervix softens.

- Nesting instinct: Some women find in the last few weeks of pregnancy they get a burst of energy and feel the need to tidy and clean; this is thought to be an inbuilt maternal urge to prepare the home for the arrival.

- Mucous plug: As the cervix softens, shortens and begins to dilate, the mucous plug that has sealed the cervix comes away. This is often referred to as a 'show' and appears as a small amount of red or brownish mucous. This can happen up to a few weeks before birth.

- Rupture of membranes (waters breaking): The amniotic sac around the baby usually ruptures at some point during labour. It can, however, happen before contractions begin. If this happens, most of these women will go into labour within 24 hours. If the waters break prior to labour, the woman must notify her midwife, who will advise her as to what she should do. Any discolouration of the waters requires urgent attention by the obstetric team to ensure the baby is not in distress.

Sometimes the mother will be asked to attend hospital, or the midwife may wait a day to see if contractions start.

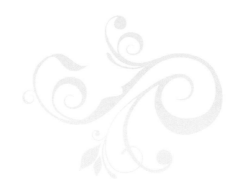

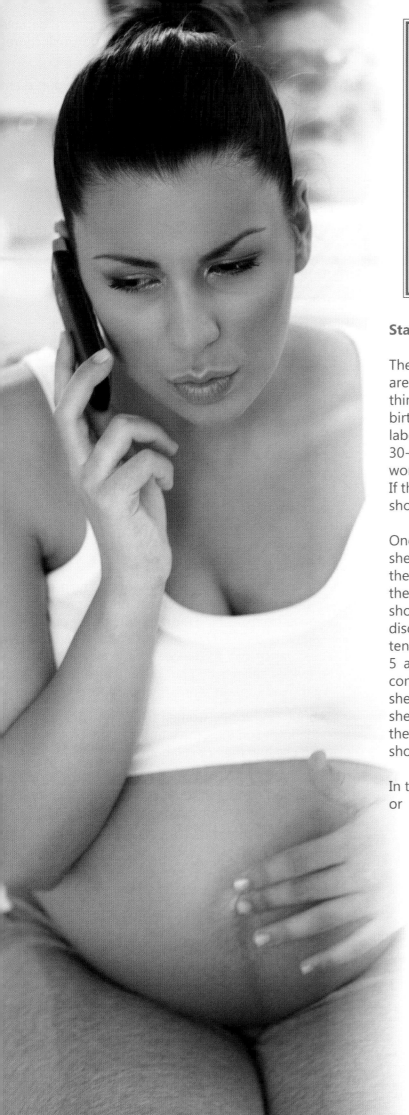

Stage 1 – Dilation of the cervix

The first stage of labour occurs when the contractions are strong and regular; the cervix opens (dilates) and thins out (effaces) to allow the baby to move into the birth canal. This is the longest of the three stages of labour. In early labour, contractions will last about 30-90 seconds and are moderately strong, but the woman will have gaps to catch her breath in between. If the woman has not had her 'show' (mucous plug), it should happen in early labour.

Once the woman is certain she is in labour she should call her midwife or hospital to let them know. Policy does vary as to when either the midwife will arrive or the woman should go into hospital, but this should have been discussed at the ante-natal classes. As the first stage tends to be a long process (on average between 5 and 15 hours), if the mother is coping with the contractions it will probably be recommended that she stays at home where it is more comfortable, as she does not need a midwife present. Remember: the more labours the woman has already had, the shorter the first stage may be.

In the UK, most women either choose a hospital birth or a planned home birth with a midwife present.

Why do women choose planned home births?

Women might choose a planned home birth for many reasons, including:

- A desire to give birth in a familiar, relaxing environment, surrounded by people of their choice.
- A desire to wear their own clothes, take a shower or bath, eat, drink and move around freely during labour.
- A desire to have greater control of some aspects of the birthing process.
- A desire to give birth without medical intervention, such as pain medication.
- Cultural or religious norms or concerns.
- Having had short, uncomplicated labours in the past.

Are there situations when a planned home birth isn't recommended?

A planned home birth isn't right for everyone. The health care provider might caution against a planned home birth if the mother:

- Has diabetes, cardiac problems, chronic hypertension, a seizure disorder or any chronic medical condition requiring close monitoring during labour.
- Previously had a caesarean section, as the new birth risks problems with the scarred area of the uterus.
- Uses tobacco or recreational drugs, which may cause withdrawal problems for the baby during labour and delivery.
- Develops a very serious pregnancy complication, such as pre-eclampsia, pre-term labour or significant anaemia, as the mother and baby require intense monitoring to prevent complications developing which will affect their wellbeing.
- Is pregnant with multiples or the baby doesn't settle into a position that allows for a headfirst delivery, which therefore risks cord prolapses, foetal distress and baby/babies getting stuck - requiring emergency caesarean section and specialised baby care.
- Is less than 37 weeks pregnant (so the baby may require special care monitoring) or more than 41 weeks pregnant, to ensure the placenta is still working well and that the baby is coping well.
- Is likely to go into precipitate labour (rapid labour of less than 2 hours) which can be dangerous and needs urgent attention to ensure no problems with foetal distress, maternal haemorrhage and perineal tears.

In the early stages of labour, the woman may be able to stay fairly active and may be able to do small chores around the house, or go for a gentle walk.

To promote comfort during early labour, your client could try:

- Taking a shower or bath.
- Listening to relaxing music.
- Having a gentle massage or reflexology.
- Slow, deep breathing exercises.
- Changing positions, walking or standing and rocking from side to side.
- Drinking water, juice or other clear liquids.
- Eating only light, healthy snacks.
- Applying ice packs or heat to her lower back.
- Attaching a TENS (transcutaneous electrical nerve stimulation) machine. A maternity TENS machine consists of a hand-held controller connected by two sets of fine leads to four sticky pads. These are placed on the back. The machine gives out little pulses of electrical energy to the skin through the pads. The pulses may give you a tingling or buzzing sensation, depending on the setting. It has buttons that the mother can use to control the frequency and strength of the pulses. There's also a boost button to press with the thumb for when she wants maximum output from the machine. This can help through each contraction.

It is unclear exactly how TENS works to help in labour. It may be that the electrical pulses prevent pain signals from reaching the brain, or that the pulses may stimulate the body to release endorphins. Despite the lack of evidence that maternity TENS provides effective pain relief in labour, most midwives support women who choose to use one.

About one in five women use TENS at some point in labour. Some mothers find it so helpful that they also use it in their next labour.

In the following text, I will discuss what will happen with a hospital birth; the same information is true for home births as well, but it will obviously be done in their own home setting.

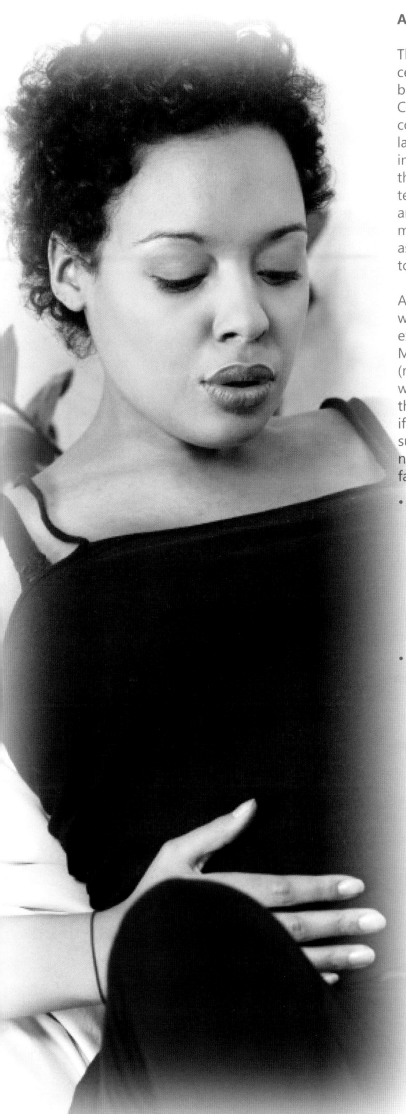

Active labour

This is the time when the real work begins! The cervix will need to become fully dilated (10cm) before the second stage of pushing begins. Contractions will get stronger, last longer and come closer together. Near the end of active labour, it might feel as though there is no break in the contractions. At this time it is essential that the mother tries to stay calm and uses breathing techniques she will have learnt either in her ante-natal classes or in ante-natal yoga. There might be increasing pressure felt in the back as well. By this time, the woman really needs to be in hospital or have a midwife present.

As the labour progresses and the pain intensifies, women can begin to get a feeling of panic, exhaustion and feel they are unable to continue. Many women go into labour with a clear idea (maybe even written into a birth plan) of what they want to happen or not during this time. Many feel they do not want any type of pain relief, but it is better if they can keep a slightly open mind as no one can be sure how they will cope with their labour. They should not be in a position where they will feel they have failed if they accept some type of pain relief such as:

- Gas and air (Entonox): This is a mixture of oxygen and nitrous oxide gas. Gas and air will not remove all the pain but it can help to reduce it and make it more bearable. Many women like it because it's easy to use and they control it themselves.

    Possible side effects – feeling light headed, nauseous, out of control.

- Injections: Another form of pain relief is the intramuscular injection of an opiate drug, such as pethidine. This can help them to relax and gain some pain relief.

    Possible side effects – feeling woozy, nauseous, poor concentration, it can make pushing harder if it is given too close to the birth. The breathing of the baby might be slightly slower and an injection will need to be given to the baby to reverse the effects.

- Epidural: An epidural is a local anaesthetic. A very small tube is placed into the lower back in the inter-space between either L2-L3, L3-L4 or L4-L5. A mixture of local anaesthetic and opioid is administered through this tube. It takes about 20 minutes to set up the epidural, and another 10 to 15 minutes for it to work. It doesn't always work perfectly at first, so may need to be adjusted. An anaesthetist is the only person who can give an epidural, so it won't be available for a home birth.

After it has been set up, the epidural can normally be topped up by a midwife. Contractions and the baby's heart will need to be continuously monitored when an epidural has been set up. For most women, an epidural gives complete pain relief. It can be helpful for women who are having a long or particularly painful labour, or who are becoming distressed.

Possible side effects – may make legs feel very heavy, can prolong second stage, headache afterwards, sore back for a couple of days or difficulty passing urine.

Active labour often lasts up to eight hours and for some women it can be even longer. For others - especially those who've had a previous vaginal delivery - active labour can be much shorter.

To promote comfort during active labour, your client could try:

- Using breathing and relaxation techniques learnt in ante-natal classes.

- TENS machine.

- Changing positions to find what is most comfortable.

- Rocking in a rocking chair or standing and rocking from side to side.

- Rolling on a birthing ball.

- Taking a warm shower or bath.

- Placing a cool, damp cloth on her forehead.

- Taking a walk, stopping to breathe through contractions.

- Having a gentle massage or reflexology between contractions.

The last part of active labour is often referred to as transition and can be particularly intense. The woman will be tired and emotional, and this is the time you are most likely to hear swearing or irrational thoughts such as 'I've had enough, I am leaving, I don't want to do this anymore'. The midwife will offer encouragement that it is nearly over.

The midwife will direct when it is time for the woman to start pushing (stage 2). Pushing too soon could cause the cervix to tear or swell, which might cause troublesome bleeding. The woman will be encouraged to pant or blow through the contractions at this time.

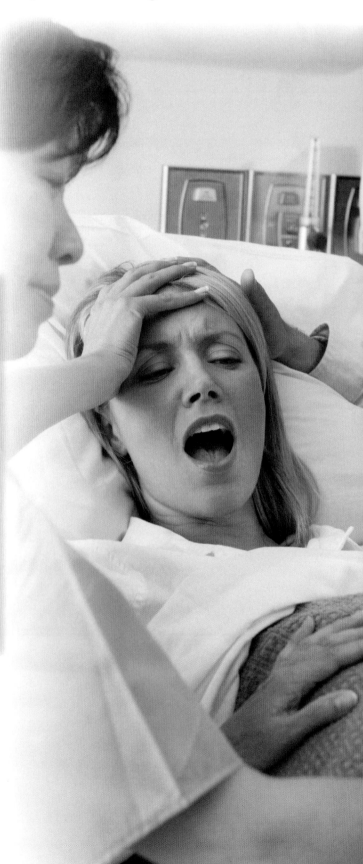

Stage 2: The birth of the baby

This is the stage where they are about to push their baby out; to see and hold their baby for the first time. After the transition phase, many women become energized, knowing the delivery is imminent. The second stage is on average around an hour, although it can be as little as 10 minutes or as long as a few hours. It often takes longer if they have had an epidural or it is their first baby.

Contractions will now be coming every two to four minutes so there is little break; there will be an urge to push but it is essential that they wait until the midwife says it is time to push; the cervix must be fully open before pushing, otherwise it can swell and become a problem. Birthing positions vary: lying backwards in a semi-supine position, sitting, lying on left side, or squatting are among the most common. It is generally felt the more upright the position the better, as gravity can help as well. This will be discussed by the midwife.

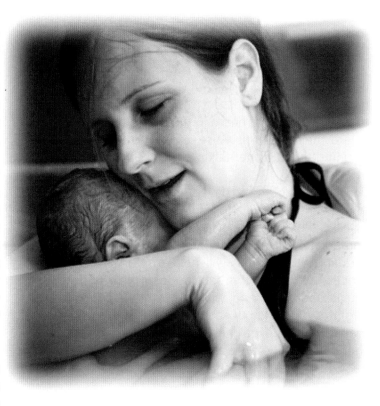

Once pushing starts, they will be encouraged to push with each contraction; the woman takes a deep breath and bears down with her abdominal muscles as she exhales. As the presenting part is delivered, they might be asked to push more gently - or not at all. Slowing down gives the vaginal tissues time to stretch rather than tear.

The first sign that the baby is about to be born is the stretching of the anus and perineum, and with each push the baby's head becomes more visible. Once the head stops slipping back but stays at the vaginal opening, it is called crowning.

As the baby is born, slow, controlled pushing is usually recommended to allow the perineum to stretch gradually and reduce the risk of tearing. The midwife may need to perform an episiotomy (a cut to the side in the perineum) if it looks like the woman will tear. An episiotomy aims to prevent and divert a damaging tear towards the anus, as a cut should heal much faster than a tear. After the baby's head is delivered, his or her airway will be cleared and the midwife will make sure the umbilical cord is free. The rest of the baby's body will follow shortly. As long as all is well, the baby will be delivered and placed onto the mother's tummy for them to meet properly for the first time.

After the birth, the umbilical cord will be clamped in two places and cut in between the two clamps; some midwives wait until the cord has stopped pulsing before they cut. At some point, the baby will be checked over to make sure all is well.

Stage 3: Delivery of the placenta

Generally, this is relatively automatic and requires little effort. After the baby is born, the uterus continues to contract and the relatively inflexible placenta will shear off from the contracting walls. The following contractions will push the placenta out.

The third stage will happen naturally, but it is common that a more active approach may be offered to speed up delivery and reduce the risk of bleeding. An injection of syntocinon or syntometrine is given in the upper leg to encourage the uterus to stay contracted and the midwife will pull gently on the cord to speed up delivery. The midwife will check that the placenta is whole; if parts are left behind, they may need to be manually removed with an epidural anaesthetic.

If the woman has chosen to breastfeed, this is encouraged as early as possible to allow early bonding. Also, as the nipple is stimulated, oxytocin is released which further promotes uterine contractions.

If they have had an episiotomy or have a tear, this is generally stitched soon after the delivery. After the birth, women can experience a wide range of emotions such as elation, excitement and exhaustion. They are likely to be hungry, thirsty and in need of a freshen up before their journey into motherhood begins.

Post-natal

The Baby

When the baby is born, they can already see (although not clearly; best vision is at a distance of 20-25cm), hear, taste, smell and sense touch. They will respond to voices they have heard in the womb and will turn to where their mother's voice is coming from. They will also find their mother talking gently to them calming.

The first few hours and days are an important time when mother and baby will hopefully bond together. As long as all is well with the baby, he or she will be placed immediately with the mother. Eye contact and cuddling at this time will help to start the bonding process, will allow the baby to learn how the mother smells and feels, and will help mother and baby to begin to get to know each other. It is also important that if there is a partner, their partner is given a fair share of bonding time as well. It is important that the baby learns to trust their parents at this early stage.

Over the first few weeks, life is mainly dominated by feeding until the baby settles into a routine. The mother needs to make the decision as to whether to breast feed or bottle feed. There is much evidence to support breastfeeding as the best option, but do remember that it is the woman's decision. There may be good reasons why they choose to bottle feed or are recommended to change to the bottle, and a mother should not be judged on her decision.

Why is breast feeding better for the baby

- Early breast milk contains colostrum, which is a thick, yellow breast milk that is made during pregnancy and just after birth. This milk is very rich in nutrients and antibodies to protect the baby.

- Breast milk changes as your baby grows: Colostrum changes into what is called mature milk. By the third to fifth day after birth, this mature breast milk has just the right amount of fat, sugar, water, and protein to help the baby continue to grow. It provides all of the nutrients and antibodies the baby needs.

- For most babies, breast milk is easier to digest than formula. The proteins in formula are generally made from cow's milk and it takes time for babies' stomachs to adjust to digesting it.

- Breast milk fights disease: the cells, hormones, and antibodies in breast milk protect babies from illness. In fact, among formula-fed babies, ear infections, asthma, respiratory infections, obesity and diarrhoea are more common.

- Reduced risks in later life: some research has shown that breastfeeding can also reduce the risk of Type 1 diabetes, dermatitis and Sudden Infant Death Syndrome (cot death). (http://www.womenshealth.gov/breastfeeding/why-breastfeeding-is-important)

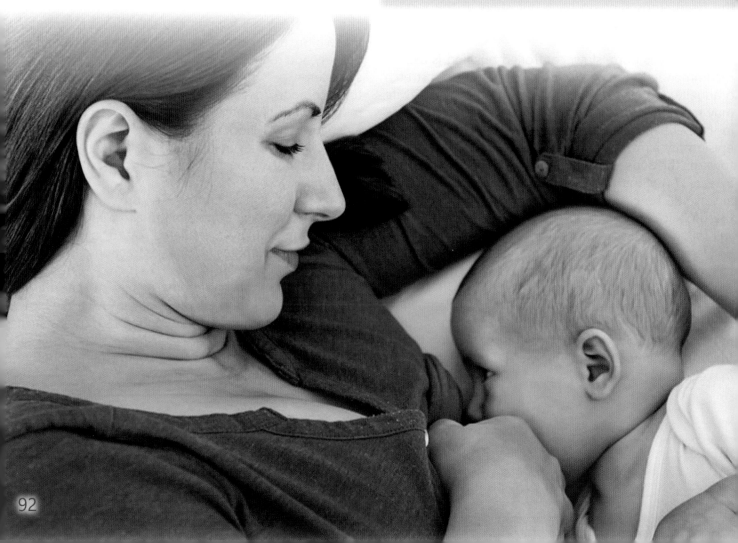

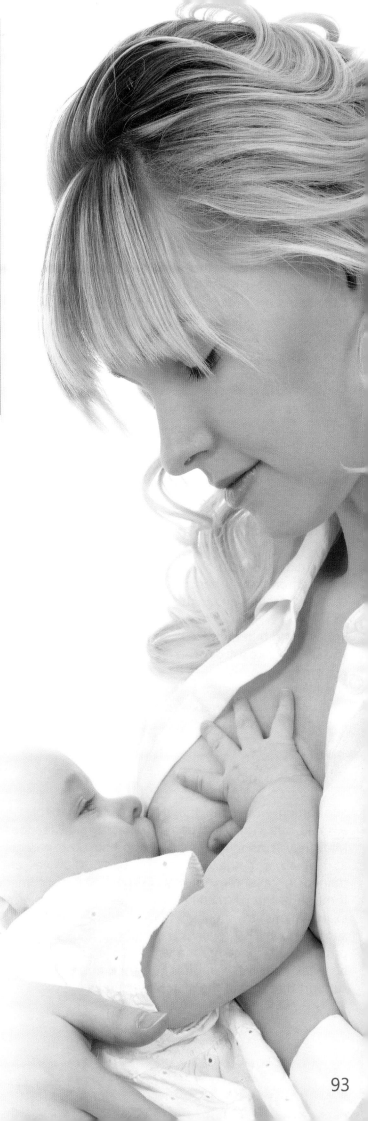

Mothers benefit from breast feeding

- Life can be easier when breastfeeding: although it may take some getting used to at first, it can make life easier once mother and baby settle into a good routine. There are no bottles to sterilize, no measuring and mixing of feeds, and breast milk is always ready to satisfy a hungry baby.

- Breast feeding can save money: Formula and feeding supplies can cost well over £1000 each year, depending on how much the baby eats.

- Breast feeding can help bonding: physical contact is important to newborns. It can help them feel more secure, warm, and comforted. Breast feeding requires a mother to take some quiet, relaxed time - which can also help bonding.

- Breast feeding can be good for the mother's health: it is linked to a lower risk of post-natal depression, and will help the uterus contract back to its pre-pregnancy state.

Information about breast feeding

The hormones that are produced during pregnancy start to change the milk ducts as they begin to get ready for breast milk production. The milk ducts increase in number and branch out with clusters of alveoli on the end.

During the pregnancy, the endocrine system will start to trigger the production of colostrum, and the milk supply will start to come within 30-40 hours of giving birth. The body doesn't produce milk before the baby is born, as levels of progesterone are too high - but once the birth is over, levels of progesterone will fall rapidly. The level of prolactin then increases (under the control of the pituitary and hypothalamus, and is also stimulated when the baby sucks) which triggers milk production. Mothers should start to breastfeed their baby as soon as possible as this will start to release prolactin and therefore trigger increased breast milk production. When the body starts producing milk, the hormone oxytocin is released by the pituitary (produced when the nipple is stimulated) and this causes the milk to be pushed out of the breast.

Oxytocin is also an important part of the bonding process. The surge of oxytocin whilst breast feeding is one of the ways that the mother falls in love with her baby, as oxytocin is also known as the love hormone.

The maternity team: *roles and responsibilities*

Mandy Forrester MA RN RN ADM PGCEA

There are various members of the health care team that are involved during the maternity journey and after the baby is born. It is important as a reflexologist to understand their roles and responsibilities; this will give you a better understanding of the care the woman is likely to be receiving and also may allow you to open up some discussions with the appropriate person if need be.

Midwives

Midwives provide most of the care for pregnant women both during their pregnancy and after their babies are born. They are trained to monitor the pregnancy and to identify any potential problems that arise, either for the mother-to-be or the baby, and will take appropriate action to minimize any potential health issues.

Most midwives work within the NHS and some work on a self-employed basis. NHS midwives work in birth centres, hospitals and in the community.

You will find that midwives work in many different ways. The style of care will depend on where you live. They may work in teams or they may be attached to GP's surgeries. Some midwives visit the women in their own homes whilst others will work from clinics. Wherever the parents-to-be are seen, the care they receive will be the same.

What does a midwife do?

Supporting women in the birthing of their babies is a small but significant part of what a midwife does. Midwifery is as much about supporting both parents, as helping with the birth of the baby. Midwives are trained to care from the day pregnancy is confirmed through to the postnatal period. They carry out clinical examinations to monitor the pregnancy and make sure the baby is growing. If a midwife finds there are problems or concerns, she will make a referral to the hospital. Midwives can offer guidance, information and support throughout the maternity journey.

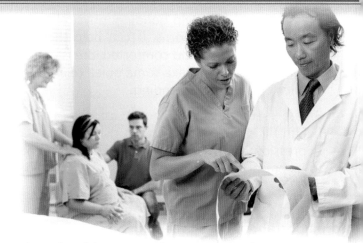

What should I expect from a midwife?

The community midwife will be informed of a new pregnancy by either the maternity service if the woman registered online or through the GP. They will then contact with the woman to get further details and plan a booking appointment for around 10 weeks into the pregnancy. At this appointment they will discuss the health and wellbeing of the woman and discuss choices and plans for the pregnancy and the birth. The woman will hold her own notes and will be provided with lots of information at this meeting.

Scans and any other appointments that are needed will also be made at this time. If the midwife finds that there are risk factors, for example diabetes, she will refer to an obstetrician.

If everything is normal and the woman fit and healthy, the midwife is responsible for care throughout the pregnancy. If the woman has risk factors such as diabetes or a small baby, the midwife works with the obstetrician to provide care.

A midwife is present at the birth of a baby whether women have their babies at home, in a birth centre or in hospital.

After birth, the community midwives will once again look after both mother and baby. Once mum and baby return home, the midwife will arrange to see both at home or in a clinic to check recovery from the labour and birth and that the baby is thriving for around the next 10 days and then a health visitor will take over the care.

If you are seeing a client for maternity reflexology, it is a good to tell the midwife so that she has a full picture of health and well being. You can either get the client to mention this or pass a note through the client introducing yourself.

Midwives' training and practice is regulated by the Nursing and Midwifery Council (NMC). You can check that the midwife is registered with the NMC and is entitled to provide midwifery care by searching the NMC register https://www.nmc.org.uk/search-the-register/

Specialist midwives

Specialist midwives are midwives who work in specific areas. Common areas for specialist midwives are diabetic care, infant feeding, teenage pregnancy, multiple births, mental health and child protection to name a few. These midwives work closely with medical specialists in their field and can provide additional information, advice and support.

Supervisors of midwives

The UK is the only place in the world where supervision of midwives occurs and it has been in place since the start of the midwifery profession in 1902.

A supervisor of midwives (SoM) is an experienced midwife who has had extra training and education to support other midwives in providing safe maternity care.

An SoM can help and support if there are any problems with care, or if the woman feels that their wishes and requests are not being considered.

For example, a supervisor of midwives can help make a plan for any specific wishes they may have such as a home birth. She is there to make sure choices are respected and that mother and baby are safe.

You can read more about supervisors of midwives and how they can help you on the NMC website:

http://www.nmc.org.uk/globalassets/siteDocuments/ NMC-Publications/NMC-Supervisor-of-midwives.pdf

Maternity Support Workers

Maternity Support Workers (MSW's) work with midwives and support midwives in providing care to pregnant women before, during and after childbirth.

Pregnant women will meet MSW's in hospital antenatal clinics, on the wards, birth centres and in the community. Their duties include doing blood tests, taking blood pressure and testing urine. Many MSW's help with classes and will give information about life with a baby.

They work on the labour wards and help midwives care for mothers and their baby immediately after birth and they may assist doctors in maternity theatre.

After a baby is born MSWs will support mothers to look after their baby. They will give advice on feeding both in the hospital and at home.

Obstetricians

An obstetrician is a trained doctor who specialises in pregnancy and childbirth.

Not all women will meet a consultant obstetrician but if there is an existing health condition or complications in pregnancy, it is likely a consultant obstetrician will play a role in planning care. The midwife will advise a woman whether there is a need to see an obstetrician at the booking visit.

Obstetricians work on the labour ward. An obstetrician may be present at the birth if help is needed for example with forceps or ventouse (a vacuum device that helps deliver the baby's head). Obstetricians are the doctors who also do caesarian sections.

Women can ask to see an obstetrician if they have any concerns that they want to discuss.

Anaesthetist

An anaesthetist is a trained doctor who specialises in providing pain relief and anaesthesia.

If a woman decides to have an epidural for pain relief during labour, an anaesthetist, who's responsible for making sure the woman can stay pain-free throughout labour, will give it.

If a caesarian section or instrumental delivery is needed, for example with forceps or ventouse (a vacuum device that helps deliver the baby's head), an anaesthetist will be responsible for the anaesthesia.

The midwife can arrange an appointment with an anaesthetist for women to discuss pain relief if there are medical or obstetric problems.

Paediatrician

A paediatrician is a trained doctor specialising in the care of babies and children.

A paediatrician may check the baby over after the birth, although this is increasingly being done by midwives who have completed training in this specialised area of care. If there are any worries about the baby's health or there has been a difficult labour, a paediatrician will be present at the birth. If there are any concerns about the baby, these can be discussed with the paediatrician. If a baby is born at home or in a birth centre the midwife or GP will check the baby.

All doctors are regulated by the General Medical Council (GMC) and you can check their credentials on the GMC website:

http://www.gmc-uk.org/doctors/register/LRMP.asp

Sonographer

A sonographer is specially trained to carry out ultrasound scans. Some midwives are trained to do scanning.

An appointment will be made with an obstetric sonographer for the 12 week and 20 week scans. Some women require scans at other stages of pregnancy to estimate the baby's growth or check its position.

Obstetric physiotherapist

An obstetric physiotherapist is specially trained to help women cope with physical changes during pregnancy, childbirth and afterwards.

An appointment will be made to see an obstetric physiotherapist if there are problems with the pelvis or back in pregnancy. Some hospitals have obstetric physiotherapists who visits the wards after the birth to advise on postnatal exercises to tone up muscles.

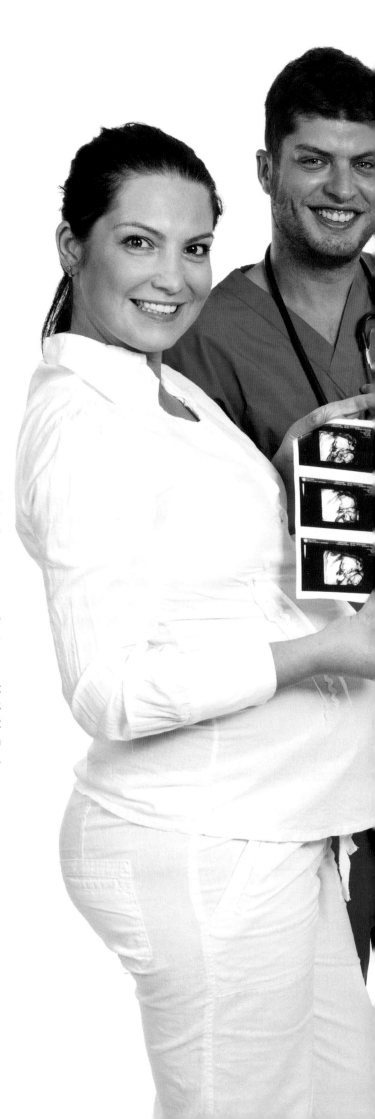

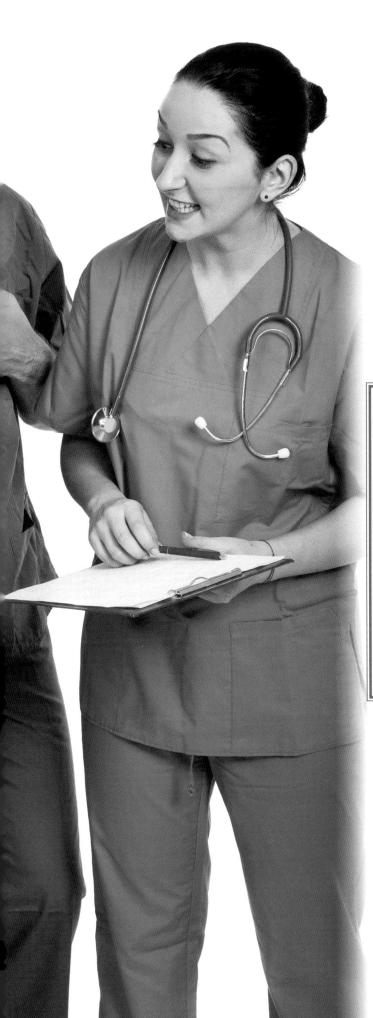

Health visitor

Health visitors are specially trained nurses who support families from pregnancy through to a child's fifth birthday.

Women may meet their health visitor before the birth of their baby and again in the first few weeks after the birth. The Health Visitor will be available to give help, support mothers to overcome any difficulties and answer any questions or concerns they may have with feeding their baby.

Students and trainee health professionals

All midwives, doctors and other health professionals need to be trained. Women may be asked if they mind if students take part in appointments, but they can say no, if they wish.

Further information:

www.nmc-uk.org

http://www.rcm.org.uk/

Mandy Forrester MA RN RN ADM PGCEA

Mandy is a qualified maternity reflexologist. She became a general nurse 1981 and a midwife in 1985.

Mandy has worked as a clinical midwife and manager in the community, in birth centres and in hospitals. She taught midwifery and has worked on various research projects. Mandy has a keen interest in regulation and worked in the United Arab Emirates where she led the team that developed midwifery regulation and registration and as a Midwifery Adviser at the Nursing and Midwifery Council.

Mandy currently works as an independent consultant on an international project and as an inspector for the Care Quality Commission.

General lifestyle advice
for pregnancy

In the following sections, we will look at lifestyle advice pertinent to each trimester. However, there are some general lifestyle factors that all pregnant women need to be aware of, and they should be encouraged to make changes if necessary.

Smoking

Smoking during pregnancy exposes a baby to carbon monoxide, which limits the baby's supply of oxygen and the delivery of nutrients. Exposure to nicotine also increases a baby's heart rate and reduces foetal breathing movements.

If a woman is still smoking when she becomes pregnant, she needs to seriously consider stopping as she is putting her baby's health at risk. There is a huge bank of evidence reporting the harm that smoking can cause to the unborn child, and here we have highlighted just some of the main concerns for smokers:

- Risk of miscarriage is significantly higher. (Ness RB, Grisso JA, Hirschinger N, et al. (February 1999). "Cocaine and tobacco use and the risk of spontaneous abortion". N. Engl. J. Med. 340 (5): 333–9.)

- Increased risk of premature birth (30% higher odds). (Centers for Disease Control and Prevention. 2009 Tobacco Use and Pregnancy: Home. http://www.cdc.gov/reproductivehealth/tobaccousepregnancy/index.htm)

- Smoking doubles a woman's risk of developing placental problems.
  (Centers for Disease Control and Prevention. 2009. Preventing Smoking and Exposure to Secondhand Smoke Before, During, and After Pregnancy. http://www.cdc.gov/chronicdisease/resources/publications/fact_sheets/smoking.htm)

- Smoking doubles the risk of low birth weight babies – babies that weigh less than 2.5kg at birth are 20 times more at risk of dying in the first year.
  (Centers for Disease Control and Prevention. 2009. Tobacco Use and Pregnancy: Home. http://www.cdc.gov/reproductivehealth/tobaccousepregnancy/index.htm)

- Infants exposed to smoke during pregnancy have a higher risk of dying of Sudden Infant Death Syndrome (SIDS, previously known as cot death). ("Patterns of Tobacco Exposure Before and During Pregnancy." Acta Obstetricia Et Gynecologica Scandinavica 89.4 (2010): 505-14. Academic Search Premier. Web. 26 April 2010. http://informahealthcare.com/doi/full/10.3109/00016341003692261

- Smoking increases the chance of birth defects such as cerebral palsy, cleft palate, asthma and many others.
  ("Patterns of Tobacco Exposure Before and During Pregnancy." Acta Obstetricia Et Gynecologica Scandinavica 89.4 (2010): 505-14. Academic Search Premier. Web. 26 April 2010. http://informahealthcare.com/doi/full/10.3109/00016341003692261

Giving up smoking can be extremely difficult. The woman should contact her GP, midwife or look at the NHS stop smoking site www.smokefree.nhs.uk for advice. Nicotine substitutes are not advisable during pregnancy. You could suggest they find out about local support groups - there is usually information in local libraries or GP surgeries.

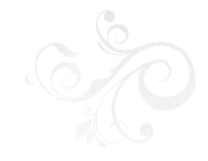

Alcohol

Alcohol can damage the developing baby, especially in the first 12 weeks of pregnancy. There is no safe level, but it is recommended that pregnant women do not have more than one unit per day (one unit = one small glass of wine, half a pint of beer/ cider, or a pub measure of spirits) and certainly not every day. Alcohol in pregnancy can lead to Foetal Alcohol Syndrome which can cause facial abnormality, heart defects, abnormal limb development and reduced intelligence in the baby.

It would of course be better if the woman did not drink at all. If the woman is a heavy drinker, they should contact their GP or midwife for advice on how to stop.

Medication

Many medications are safe during pregnancy but it is also well known that some drugs can affect the developing baby. If the woman is on medication for a medical condition like diabetes, thyroid disease, high blood pressure, or epilepsy, then they should consult their GP as soon as possible to discuss their treatment.

Recent studies have shown that over-the-counter painkillers like Ibuprofen and Aspirin should not be used in pregnancy. Any over-the-counter medication should be discussed with the pharmacist first to check that it is safe to use in pregnancy.

Exercise

Everyone should exercise for 30 minutes at least five days a week and this is the same in pregnancy. Exercise strengthens the whole body and allows toxins to be dealt with by helping to move lymph around the lymphatic system.

If a woman has been taking regular exercise, there will be benefits to her throughout pregnancy; especially later in pregnancy and during labour when extra demands are made of the body. Aerobic exercise like swimming, cycling, walking or dancing are ideal ways to prepare the body for labour. Ante-natal yoga exercises may also be helpful. Midwives should be able to advise your client further.

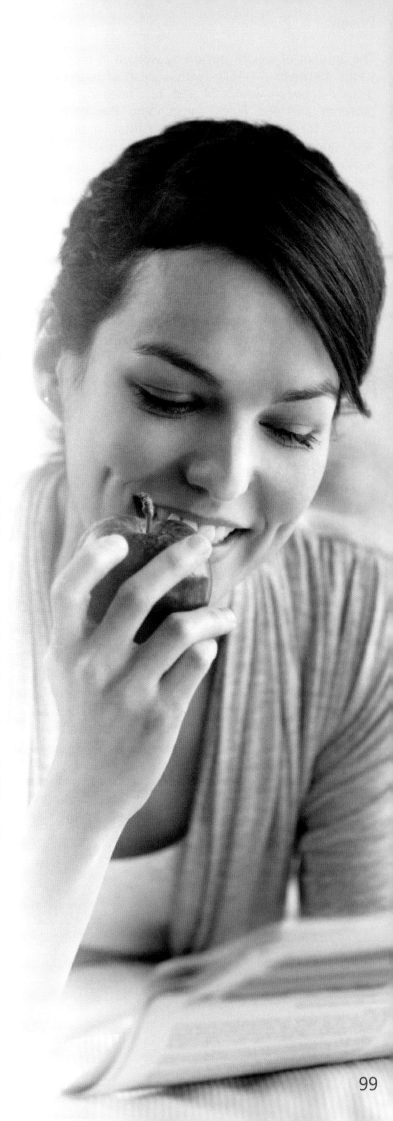

Weight

The amount of weight put on by women in pregnancy varies between 11-16kg with the most rapid gain usually between weeks 24 and 32. The baby, uterus, placenta and the fluids surrounding the baby will account for more than half of the total weight gain. Also, during this time, blood volume increases and fat is stored in preparation for breast feeding. If women put on more than this during pregnancy, it can lead to extra issues later in pregnancy such as backache, varicose veins etc.

Nutrition

The midwife will go through general nutrition with your client, but below we have highlighted the foods that should be avoided and those that should be encouraged during pregnancy.

Foods to avoid:

- Seafood high in mercury: e.g. swordfish, shark, king mackerel. However, fish that contain a little mercury e.g. tuna (including tinned), salmon, pollock, cod, tilapia may be eaten - but no more than twice a week.

- Raw or undercooked meat, poultry, eggs and fish – as this increases the risk of serious bacterial infection.

- Unpasteurised cheeses such as brie, feta, camembert and blue cheeses, as there is a risk of gastric infections.

During pregnancy, the basic principles of healthy eating remain the same - plenty of fruits, vegetables, whole grains and lean protein. A balanced diet will ensure that all vitamins and minerals are available to both mother and baby.

In addition to making healthy food choices, taking a daily pregnancy vitamin supplement (ideally starting three months before conception), can help ensure that correct levels of vitamins and nutrients are achieved.

Foods to encourage

- Folate and folic acid: helps prevent neural tube defects, as well as serious abnormalities of the brain and spinal cord. Lack of folate in a pregnancy diet may also increase the risk of low birth weight and pre-term delivery. The synthetic form of folate found in supplements and fortified foods is known as folic acid.

  How much: 600 micrograms of folate or folic acid a day before conception and throughout pregnancy. Most woman choose to take a folic acid supplement to ensure they achieve the correct amount.

  Good natural sources: Fortified cereals are great sources of folic acid. Leafy green vegetables, citrus fruits, and dried beans and peas are good sources of naturally occurring folate.

- Calcium: Both mother and baby need calcium for strong bones and teeth. Calcium also helps circulatory, muscular and nervous systems run normally.

  How much: 800 milligrams a day.

  Good natural sources: Dairy products are the richest sources of calcium, but there are other good sources as well such as sesame seeds, soya, tofu, flax seeds, almonds and brazil nuts.

- Iron: for new cell and hormone formation.

  Iron constitutes a large part of haemoglobin (oxygen carrying protein in red blood cells) and as blood volume may double in pregnancy, the demand for iron is greatly increased. It is not uncommon for women to become anaemic during pregnancy, so foods rich in iron are to be encouraged.

  N.B. Vitamin C enhances iron absorption, so citrus fruit or citrus fruit juice should be taken when foods containing iron are eaten.

  How much: 15 milligrams a day.

  Good sources: red meat, poultry, fish, green vegetables, pasta, grains, nuts, eggs and fortified cereals.

Common tests *in* *pregnancy*

Ultrasound scans

This is a painless and harmless scan that uses a probe that moves over the surface of the abdomen: high-frequency sound waves pass through the abdomen into the womb. The sound is reflected back and this creates a picture, which is seen on a screen. It can be very exciting for the potential parents to see a picture of their own baby moving about.

The ultrasound pictures should be explained to the woman as the probe moves around, and it is usually possible to have a picture of the baby for the parents to take home; however, there is often a charge for this.

Heartbeat scan - 6-10 weeks

This is an ultrasound scan that, although not routinely offered to all women, is often used for women who have undergone fertility treatment or have had a history of miscarriage. It is also used for women who are experiencing bleeding or abdominal pain to rule out ectopic pregnancy (where the foetus implants and grows in the fallopian tube rather than the uterus).

The scan is usually done vaginally as an abdominal scan will not be able to pick up the heartbeat at this early stage. This means a probe is inserted into the vagina to be able to pick up the heartbeat. Although this may cause worry, there is no evidence that the probe can harm the foetus. The scan will only be able to pick up the heartbeat, as it is too early to check if the foetus is healthy.

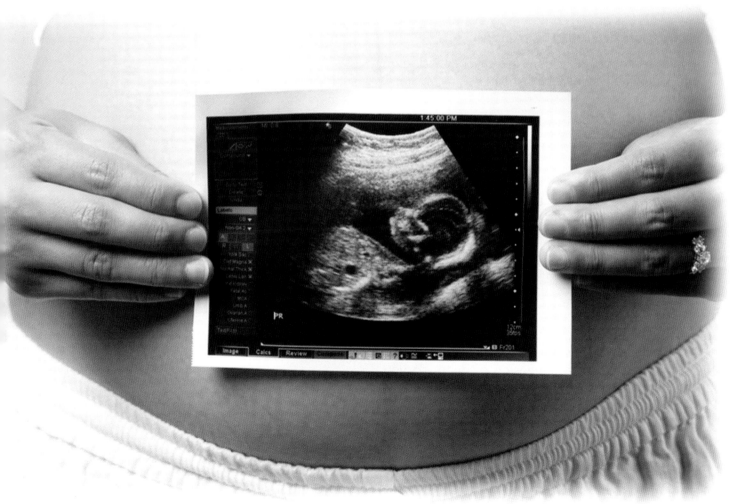

Early dating scan and Nuchal Translucency screening - 10-14 weeks

The first routine ultrasound scan offered to all women is the dating scan, which is usually an abdominal ultrasound scan. This scan will be able to:

* Ensure the foetus has implanted in the uterus.

* Establish an accurate due date.

* Check if it is a single or multiple pregnancy.

* Check the uterus and ovaries are healthy.

At this time, all women will be offered a Nuchal Translucency (NT) test which assesses the risk of Down's syndrome. It is the woman's choice as to whether or not she has this. If she agrees to the NT test, this is a simple measurement of the nuchal space that is done during the scan. The nuchal space is a special fluid-filled area at the back of the neck; if this is thicker than average, the risk of Down's syndrome is increased and the woman will be offered further tests e.g. serum testing and possibly amniocentesis.

It is important to realise that the NT test does not confirm whether or not the foetus has Down's syndrome, but only estimates the risk e.g. 1 in 1000, 1 in 100, 1 in 10 etc. It is then the woman's decision as to whether she wants further tests.

Anomaly scan – 18-20 weeks

As the foetus has grown considerably by this stage, the scan is far more detailed. This scan checks:

* Foetal anatomy – all organs are checked including the brain and spinal cord, heart, stomach, face, kidneys, limbs.

* Growth rate.

* Amount of amniotic fluid.

* Location of the placenta.

* Gender of the foetus – if the parents want to know!

There may be further scans offered if there are multiple pregnancies or concerns about the pregnancy.

3-D and 4-D scans

Some women are now choosing to pay to have a 3-D or 4-D scan, which gives amazingly clear images. The 3-D scan adds the extra dimension of depth so you can actually see the shape of the baby's face and body. The 3-D pictures can be seen on a screen and are then put onto a CD for the mother to take home.

The 4-D scan adds the further dimension of time, giving a moving 3D image of the baby. The video is then put onto a DVD for the mother to take home.

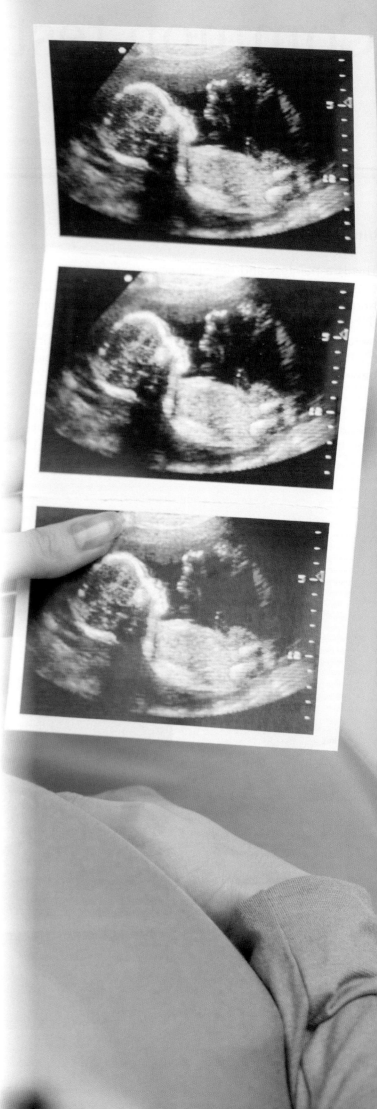

MATERNAL BLOOD TESTS

Early blood test

Early in the pregnancy, the mother will have blood tests to test for:

- Blood group: in case a transfusion is needed during pregnancy or labour.

- Rhesus factor status: if the mother is Rhesus negative and her baby is Rhesus positive, the mother's body can develop antibodies if the two bloods mix (e.g. during the birth). This could cause problems in subsequent pregnancies if the baby is Rhesus positive. The antibodies that the mother produced in the first pregnancy can destroy any subsequent Rhesus positive foetus.

  If the mother is Rhesus negative, she will be given injections of anti-D, which will prevent the mother making antibodies.

- Full blood count: This will check the levels of red blood cells, white blood cells and platelets. The red blood cell count in particular is important to check for anaemia, which is common in pregnancy as blood volume increases. Blood tests to check the full blood count will be carried out several times during the pregnancy to check for anaemia.

- Rubella (German Measles): Most adult women are immune to this virus, but if they are not immune, they should try to avoid coming into contact with children who have this.

- Hepatitis B: This is the most common viral liver infection, usually transferred through infected blood e.g. contaminated needles or having unprotected sex with an infected person. If the mother is infected, the baby will be given a vaccination immediately after the birth.

- HIV: All women in the UK are now routinely offered a blood test for HIV, as it is possible to be infected and not realise it. There are now many ways in which an unborn baby can be protected from catching HIV from an infected mother.

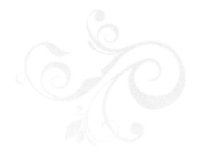

- Screening tests: All pregnant women should be offered a screening blood test for genetic abnormalities in their baby, such as Down's syndrome. One of the most accurate tests is the combined screening test. This consists of blood tests and a nuchal translucency scan carried out at the end of the first trimester.

  This combined test is now recommended in the UK. It gives a more reliable risk rating as to whether the baby may have a problem, but is not available in all NHS Trusts.

Other blood tests that may be offered in pregnancy

- Sickle cell anaemia and thalassaemia: this will only be offered if there is a chance that the mother has one of these disorders. These blood-cell disorders can cause anaemia and can be passed on to the baby.

  In the UK, sickle cell disorders are more common in people of African and African-Caribbean descent. Thalassaemia is more common in people of Asian, Mediterranean, Middle Eastern or African descent.

- Glucose Tolerance Test (GTT): There is a form of diabetes called gestational diabetes, which is common in pregnancy (this is discussed in more detail later). The policy for whether this is carried out routinely or not depends on the NHS Trust. Some women will have a routine GTT between 24 and 28 weeks. Other Trusts will only offer it if sugar is picked up on a routine urine test.

GENETIC TESTING

Depending on age, family history, results from blood screening and some other factors, some women may be offered (or may ask for) genetic testing to detect certain genetic conditions. For this, a cell needs to be taken from the foetus for individual chromosomes to be studied. The most common chromosomal abnormality is Down's syndrome, but other hereditary conditions can be detected such as cystic fibrosis, muscular dystrophy, sickle cell disease, Huntington's disease, haemophilia etc.

Having genetic screening comes with a risk of miscarriage; each woman will have to decide if this risk is worth taking in order to identify possible genetic problems.

CHORIONIC VILLUS SAMPLING (CVS)

This is a test which takes cells from the placenta, which has the same genetic make-up as the developing foetus. The main advantage over amniocentesis is that it can be carried out earlier in pregnancy. CVS is usually done between 10 and 13 weeks and the sample can be taken in two ways - either transabdominal (a hollow needle is inserted through the abdomen), or transcervical (where a flexible sampling device is inserted via a catheter guided by ultrasound.

The risk of miscarriage with CVS is approximately 1:1000. Vaginal bleeding is common after this procedure; this should only be reported to the healthcare provider if this lasts for more than three days or the woman develops a fever, as this may indicate an infection.

Results are usually ready in about 7 days.

AMNIOCENTESIS

This test involves withdrawing amniotic fluid which contains cells from the baby. This is usually done between 15 to 20 weeks, but cannot be used for all genetic abnormalities. A needle is inserted into the amniotic fluid guided by an ultrasound scan, and approximately 20ml of fluid is withdrawn.

The risk of miscarriage with amniocentesis is the same as with CVS - 1:1000. There is often some cramping after the procedure and the woman should rest.

Results are usually ready within 2 weeks.

FOETAL BLOOD SAMPLING

This is where foetal blood is withdrawn from the umbilical cord, and is usually performed after 18 weeks of pregnancy. The advantage of this test is that results are usually ready within three days so it tends to be used if a fast result is critical e.g. concerns about foetal infection or foetal anaemia. The procedure is carried out in the same way as CVS but the needle is inserted into the umbilical cord not the placenta.

The risk with this test is much higher, with between 1 and 2 per hundred resulting in miscarriage.

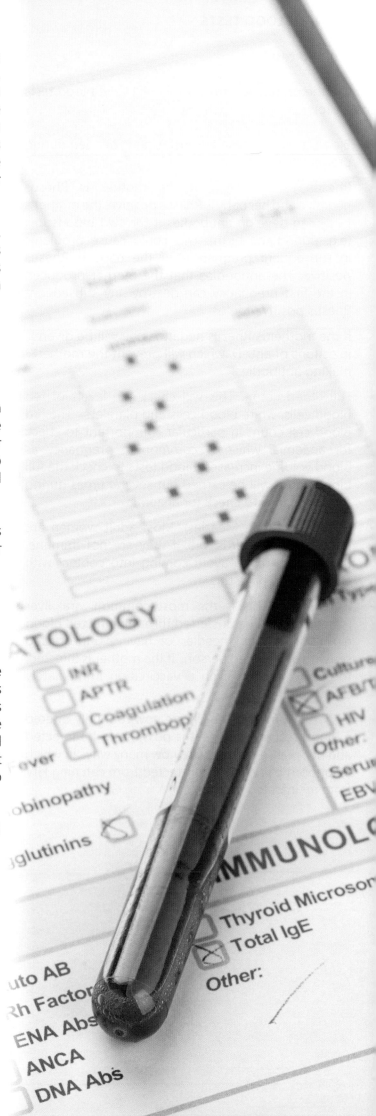

TESTS AT THE ANTENATAL APPOINTMENTS

Most women will be seen regularly from about 10 weeks onwards by a midwife, and sometimes a doctor. How often a woman is seen depends upon her medical needs and where she lives. As long as the pregnancy is straightforward, there will be approximately 10 ante-natal appointments around 16 weeks, 25 weeks, 28 weeks, 31 weeks, 34 weeks, 36 weeks, 38 weeks, 40 weeks and 41 weeks (if they have not had the baby by then).

There are some tests that will be carried out every time they have an ante-natal appointment:

- Weight: to check that weight gain is within the expected range. If a woman is gaining too much weight, this may indicate gestational diabetes and if a woman is not gaining enough weight, the growth of the baby will be checked.

- Blood pressure: This is an essential part of ante-natal care as a high blood pressure may be an indication of pre-eclampsia (discussed later). This can be life threatening if left untreated.

- Urine test: this will look for urine infection, protein (which may indicate pre-eclampsia), and glucose (in which case a glucose tolerance test may be used to check for gestational diabetes). The test is usually analysed immediately, as the midwife can dip a special strip into the urine, giving results within a couple of minutes. Occasionally a sample will be sent to a laboratory to investigate in more detail.

- Growth and foetal position: at each visit, the healthcare provider will palpate the abdomen and measure the fundal height (distance from the pelvic bone to the top of the uterus) to estimate the growth of the foetus. If there is concern that the foetus is growing too fast or too slowly, an ultrasound scan is likely to be booked.

- Heartbeat: most midwives carry a hand-held Sonicaid fetal heart monitor, which amplifies the baby's heartbeat so the mother can hear it. The baby's heart rate is much faster than an adults and is usually between 120 beats and 160 beats per minute (BPM).

- Movement: The midwife will also ask if the foetus is moving. Movement is not generally felt until after 18 weeks, when it can feel like a butterfly. As the baby grows, movements become bigger and stronger, until space becomes limited as the birth approaches and the movements become less frequent.

This is only a guide as to normal tests that are carried out. These will vary depending on the area in which the woman lives and how the pregnancy is progressing. Remember: if your client has any concerns, they should contact their healthcare provider - even if it's in between appointments.

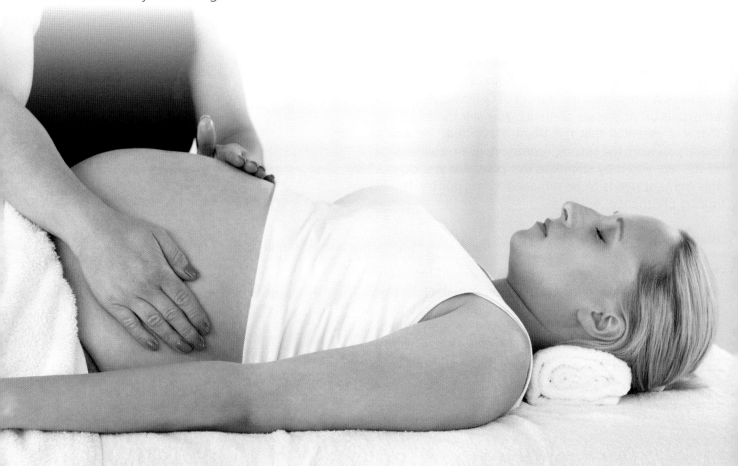

General reflexology information *relating to pregnant and post natal women*

In each section of the following chapter, there are suggestions for reflexology points or techniques that should be worked to support women with different health issues. There are a few basic principles that are useful to cover at this point.

Spleen 6 should not be worked

In the guidelines, it states that there is an acupressure point called Spleen 6 - this should not be worked during maternity. It is found 2 ½ fingers up from the medial malleolus (ankle bone). This is a rough guide, as it is actually 2 ½ of your client's fingers; so if your fingers are larger or smaller than your client's, then it may be 2-3 fingers up from the malleolus.

It is called Spleen 6 as it is the 6th acupressure point on the spleen meridian, which originates on the big toe and moves up the inside of the leg. This point, if stimulated, frees blood stasis from the uterus and produces a downward movement of Qi (energy), causing an expulsion of uterine contents. You can therefore see that it is essential that this point is avoided. Be aware that if you work the chronic reproductive area either side of the leg, you may stimulate this point – if you do use this move, it needs to be removed from your treatment during pregnancy.

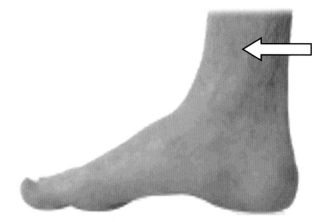

Spleen 6

Bladder 60 – caution!

This is another acupressure point you should be aware of. It is located anterior to the lateral maleolus. This point is used to speed up labour, and again should not be used during maternity unless you are treating a client during labour and have been specifically trained to use this acupressure point.

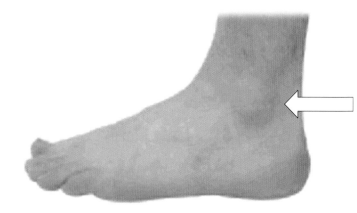

Bladder 60

Concentrating on a reflex point or area

In the following chapter, there are recommended reflex points or areas that I have suggested you concentrate on for different symptoms. This can mean you spend longer on the reflex, work it from different angles or revisit it several times during your treatment. You can try out different ways to see which you feel works best for you.

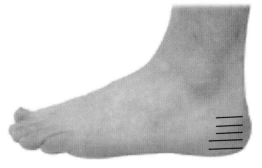

Pelvic area (lateral)

Pelvic area

We will refer to working the pelvic area with knuckles or fingers; this refers to the back area of the heel. Massaging this area can help ease tension in the area and is useful to remember when treating pregnant women - it can be tender, so treat gently to begin with.

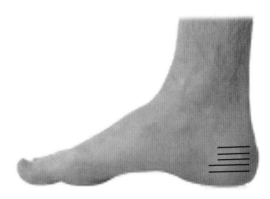

Pelvic area (medial)

Toe triangle

You will see that the term Toe Triangle is frequently mentioned. This term refers to pituitary, hypothalamus and pineal reflexes. Although pineal can be useful for circadian rhythms and sleep disturbance, it is often only the pituitary and hypothalamus that need to have more time spent working them. The reason I will refer to working the toe triangle is because I have trained many qualified reflexologists in Maternity Reflexology, and it soon came to my attention that the hypothalamus and pineal reflexes are often taught in different positions (i.e. just above pituitary is referred to as hypothalamus by some and as the pineal by others). If you look at different foot charts, you will also see these referred to in different positions. So rather than debating which is correct, it seemed sensible to include them as one sequence (Toe Triangle) to ensure all are covered.

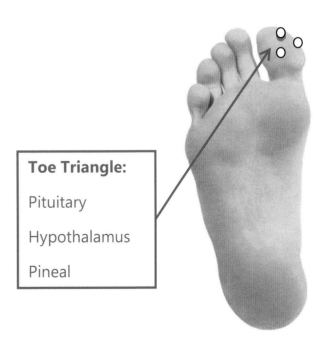

Toe Triangle:

Pituitary

Hypothalamus

Pineal

Linking

For further information on linking, please see page 60 and Appendix 2 on p151 - 152.

Unwind technique

Some reflexologists also hold the belief that if you wish to calm a reflex (e.g. stomach if there is nausea, or adrenals if anxious) the reflex should be gently massaged using an anti-clockwise movement on the right soles and clockwise on the left (thumbs, fingers or knuckles can be used to make small circular movements over the reflex point that you wish to calm). Likewise, if you wish to stimulate a reflex, you can use deeper pressure to stimulate the reflex followed by clockwise massage over the area on the right sole, and anti-clockwise on the left.

Open Spine technique

This movement opens up and helps the function of the Central Nervous System. Taking one foot at a time, place both thumbs at the C1 (the very top of the neck) reflex. In tandem, stroke downwards and outwards in small, sweeping movements along the length of the spinal reflexes. Imagine the nerve plexi fanning out from the spinal cord; if you follow the same pattern with your strokes, ending up with your thumbs perpendicular to the spinal reflexes at the edges of the foot, you will have the correct movement. Alternatively, use the side of your thumb to rub across the spine, place the side of your thumb on each vertebrae and rub across the spine - forwards and backwards (plantar to dorsal and then dorsal to plantar), so you are working across the spine rather than along it.

Spinal twist

This is a great move for opening a treatment with. Taking one foot at a time, place both hands curved fully over the top part of the medial aspect of the foot, with the uppermost hand over the C1 reflex. This will mean that the palms of your hands rest over the spinal reflexes, whilst the fingers and thumbs curve around the foot. With a wringing motion similar to unscrewing the lid from a jar, work along the spinal reflexes to loosen them throughout.

Endocrine balance

This technique was developed by Susanne Enzer in her book Reflexology: a Tool for Midwives, published in 2000. This technique can be found on pages 3-30 and is particularly helpful in balancing hormones; therefore, it is ideally suited for use during pregnancy, labour and post-natally when the body is needing to adapt to huge changes in hormone levels. The method for this technique is outlined below with kind permission from Susanne Enzer of the Maternity Reflexology Consortium.

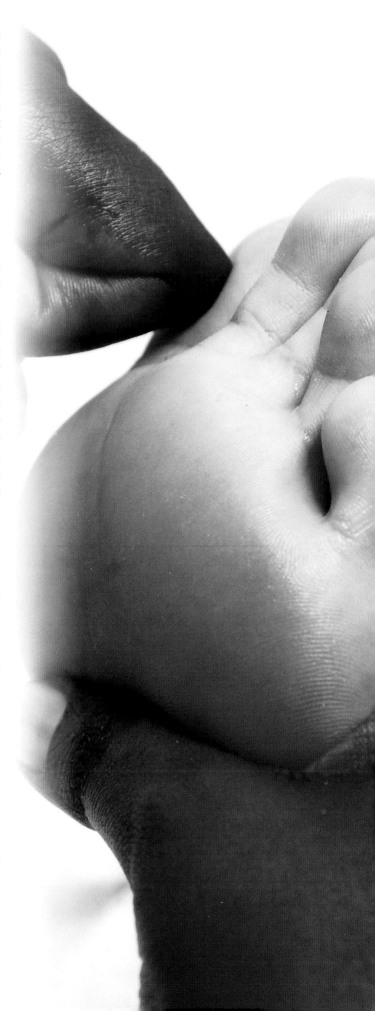

Method

1. Identify the endocrine system reflexes. Work both feet simultaneously.

2. Gently stimulate these reflex zones:

   Hypothalamus – use the pad of the thumb. Press gently but firmly into the reflex. Bounce gently on the reflexes

   Pineal gland – use the 'thumb walking' area of the thumb. Thumb walk on the spot

   Pituitary gland - use the 'thumb walking' area of the thumb. Thumb walk on the spot

   Thyroid and parathyroid glands – use the 'thumb walking' area of the thumb. Thumb walk the reflex zones

   Thymus – use the 'thumb walking' area of the thumb. Thumb walk and tap the reflex zones

   Pancreas - use the 'thumb walking' area of the thumb. Thumb walk the reflex zones – lateral to medial

   Adrenal gland - use the pad of the thumb. Press gently into the reflex. Bounce gently on the reflexes until you feel a response

   Ovaries – Place the thumb on the direct ovary reflex and third finger on the indirect ovary reflex. Make a pinch type movement of thumbs and fingers

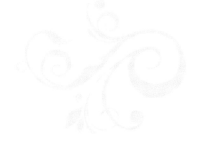

Method (contd)

Connect the reflex zones of the endocrine system together by stroking from:

- Ovaries to adrenals
- Adrenals to pancreas
- Pancreas to thymus
- Thymus to thyroid and parathyroid
- Thyroid to pituitary
- Pituitary to pineal
- Pineal to hypothalamus
- Balance the energy – repeat the sequence. Hold each reflex in turn until the energies feel the same or for no longer than 2 minutes

Connect the reflex zones of the endocrine system (as used at the top of this box)

If the energy does not balance in time, complete the endocrine balance then return to the reflex zone which needs attention

Method © Suzanne Enzer: reproduced by kind permission

In summary

It is important as a reflexologist who is treating a maternity client that you have an understanding of maternal and foetal development, as well as suitable reflexology techniques. Remember: you are not responsible for maternity care and this needs to be made clear to the client so they do not have unrealistic expectations of you.

The following chapter will look at the three trimesters, labour and post-natal in terms of:

- Common symptoms and general lifestyle advice
- Adapting reflexology to meet the client's needs

For pictures to help you with this technique, also see pages 60 - 62.

Common symptoms, lifestyle advice and *for the three trimesters*

Common symptoms and lifestyle advice for the first trimester

Morning sickness

This is very common in the first trimester; in fact the majority of pregnant women feel nauseous or sick in the early stages of their pregnancy (1) and typically this will improve after the first trimester. Nausea can begin as early as three weeks after conception. It is most common in the mornings, but can strike at any time of day and occasionally can be constant, with very little respite from feeling sick. This can go along with a heightened and altered sense of smell, which means some odours such as cooking food, perfume, smoke, etc may cause waves of nausea in early pregnancy - so remember to keep your treatment room free of strong smells.

The cause of nausea during pregnancy isn't clear, some thoughts are that:

- Morning sickness generally starts at the same time as levels of hCG rise - so it may just be a symptom of rising levels of this hormone, which is required for a healthy pregnancy.

- It may be nature's way of helping to protect the foetus by:

  ➢ Reducing exposure to potentially dangerous substances. Many women will go off caffeine drinks, alcohol and smoking, which would be potentially harmful to the foetus.

  ➢ Encouraging the pregnant woman to eat foods that contain required nutrients for a healthy pregnancy.

➢ Producing rising levels of oestrogen and progesterone: however, these also slow the action of the stomach down. This may cause nausea.

There are a number of things that a pregnant woman can do to lessen the symptoms of nausea. There is little proven evidence to support these suggestions, but it is worth your clients trying the following:

- Eating small, frequent meals throughout the day.

- Having a dry cracker or biscuit before they get out of bed in the morning.

- Avoiding foods or smells that make their nausea worse.

- Choosing foods that are low in fat and easy to digest.

- Drink plenty of fluids as becoming dehydrated may the nausea worse.

- Smell citrus fruits, especially fresh cut lemon.

- Try drinking ginger ale or ginger tea.

- Try motion sickness bands.

References

(1) www.nct.org.uk/pregnancy/nausea-and-vomiting-pregnancy

Fatigue

This is also a common symptom in the first trimester. During early pregnancy, the high levels of progesterone can cause tiredness. There are also extra demands being put on the body and these may lower blood sugar levels, increasing exhaustion.

To try and combat fatigue, women can try:

- Eating small regular meals, making sure they are getting enough iron and protein.

- Resting as much as possible. This can be particularly hard in the first trimester as women are often still working.

- Taking exercise, such as a brisk walk, even if they don't feel like it, as it can help energy levels.

- Avoiding caffeine, as it can cause drops in energy levels.

- Accepting help if it is offered.

Breast tenderness

This is one of the earliest signs of pregnancy, starting at around week 4-6 and continuing throughout the first trimester. This is due to the increase in oestrogen and progesterone causing increased blood flow and changes in the breast tissue. This may make the breasts feel swollen, sore, tingly and unusually sensitive to touch.

At around 6 to 8 weeks, the breasts will start to get bigger and they will continue to grow throughout your pregnancy. The other noticeable change is that nipples and areolas begin to darken due to the increase in hormones.

It may be helpful for a client experiencing breast tenderness to:

- Wear a supportive cotton bra, which may be more comfortable without an underwire.

- Wear a cotton sports bra to bed if their breasts are tender at night.

- Discuss the tenderness with their partner as even a hug can hurt.

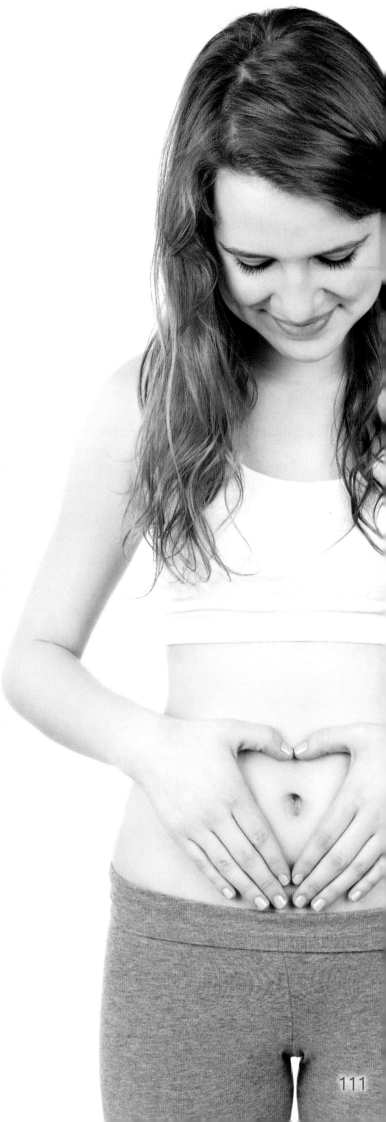

Heartburn and constipation

These can also be an issue during the first trimester, as the high level of oestrogen slows down the whole digestive tract, including the emptying of the stomach and passage through the intestines. This will allow more nutrients to be absorbed, but can also cause heartburn and indigestion.

It may be helpful for a client experiencing heartburn or constipation to try and:

- Eat small, frequent meals.
- Avoid fried foods, carbonated drinks, citrus fruits or juices and spicy foods.
- Include plenty of fibre in their diet, to prevent or relieve constipation.
- Drink plenty of water.
- Get regular physical activity.

Dizziness

Feeling light-headed during the first trimester can also be an issue, as the high level of progesterone relaxes the walls of the blood vessels, causing the vessels to dilate and blood pressure to drop - this can cause a lightheaded feeling or dizziness. Stress, fatigue and hunger also may play a role. Dizziness can continue throughout pregnancy for different reasons which we will look at in the following sections.

It may be helpful for a client experiencing dizziness to try and:

- Avoid prolonged standing.
- Rise slowly after lying or sitting down.
- Sit or lie down if they're standing when dizziness hits.
- Eat small, regular meals to keep blood sugar levels constant.

Emotional Issues

With all the hormonal changes that are happening this is a time where many women feel they are on an emotional rollercoaster. Even if a woman is delighted about the pregnancy, there will still be areas of emotional stress in her life.

Expectant mothers may have concerns about the pregnancy, including worries about the birth, the baby's health, and how they will adapt to motherhood. There may also be concerns about the financial stress of raising a child, how they will balance work and motherhood, how the baby will affect the relationship with their partner and whether they will be a good parent.

It is important to reassure the 'mother-to-be' that all these feelings, mood swings and bouts of tears are quite normal. She must feel able to talk about how she is feeling - most importantly, encourage her to talk to her partner, family and close friends. As a reflexologist you are just there to listen, empathise and not to judge. Also be prepared for the mood swings; her mood may vary from week to week or even within one treatment session, and remember to always have that box of tissues to hand!

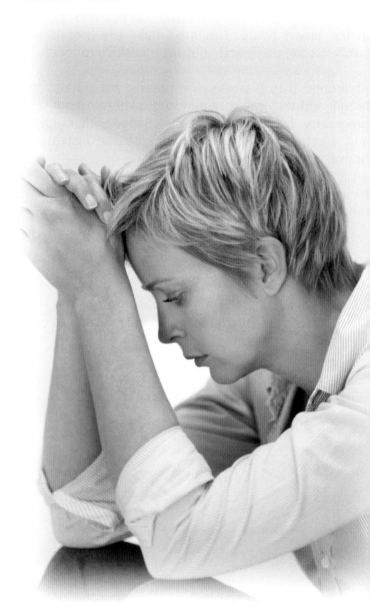

Reflexology in the First Trimester

As mentioned, it is essential that you read the Association of Reflexologists' information sheet for treating during pregnancy in full (pages 73-76), but certainly, if you have any concerns or doubts with any of the following, you should not treat in the first trimester:

- Do you have the relevant experience? (If you are unsure, then check the maternity thermometer - Appendix 1 on page 150).

- Have you provided your client with all relevant information, discussed and managed her expectations and answered any questions she had?

- Are you and your client completely happy with providing and receiving the treatment respectively?

- If the client were to miscarry following their reflexology session, would you be able to deal with the client appropriately, and be able to emotionally cope yourself with the inevitable upset and self-questioning that will follow?

- Does the client have a history of miscarriage or unstable pregnancy? Such is the level of caution required in these circumstances that it is recommended that only reflexologists with a depth of knowledge, understanding and experience in this area should even contemplate taking on clients in this category. To add to this, it is recommended that your client should contact their doctor regarding receiving reflexology. Following this, all the considerations concerning contraindications and cautions apply, in particular the ability of the reflexologist to cope with any eventuality.

Dos and don'ts

- Do focus on the client's health and any symptoms they may be experiencing.

- Do take extra care to ensure client comfort.

- Do allow extra time between ending the session and the client standing up.

- Do research and understand your subject.

- Do attend a CPD workshop/course on pregnancy.

- Don't exceed your training and experience.

- Don't treat pregnancy as an illness.

- Don't have the room too warm.

- Do be aware of smells in the treatment room - some pregnant women have a very sensitive sense of smell!

- Don't use any essential oils unless you are qualified to do so. This includes includes being aware of the therapeutic level of aromatherapy oils in any wax or cream that you use.

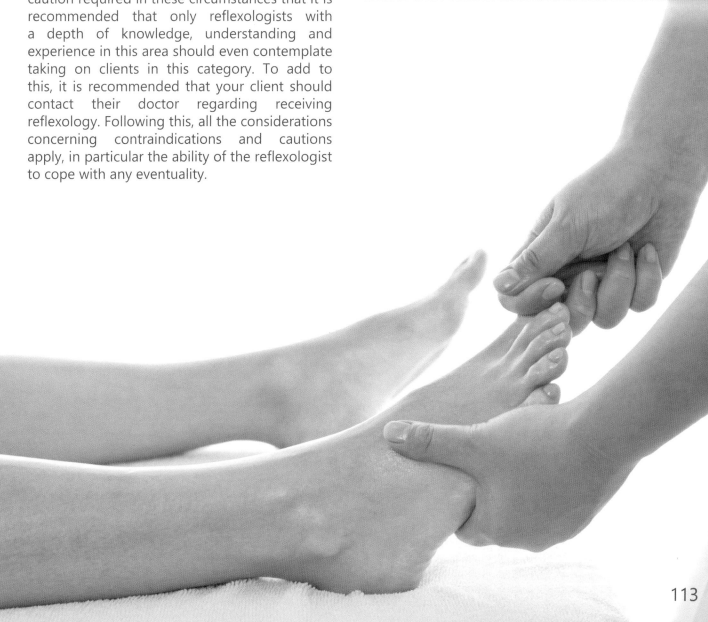

Are there any reflex points that should be avoided?

There are no actual reflexology points that need to be avoided with maternity clients; however, there is one acupuncture point that does need to be avoided in pregnancy as it would in Traditional Chinese Medicine. This is Spleen 6, which was discussed in the Introduction and on page 106.

Just as a reminder, this is located on the medial side of the ankle, about two-and-a-half of the client's finger widths up from the medial malleolus. As this is not a universally taught reflex point that is part of a regular reflexology session, there should be no reason to work on this reflex. Be aware, however, if you work the chronic pelvic area by stimulating up either side of the ankle bone and calf muscle, you will in fact be working over Spleen 6, so this move should not be used until post 37 weeks.

Some schools teach that the ovaries, uterus, pituitary and thyroid reflexes should be avoided at all times throughout pregnancy. Current information suggests that there is no reason to avoid these reflexes, but neither is it recommended that you should specifically work into these areas unless you have had training.

How often should I see the client?

This should be discussed with each client, but certainly in the first trimester it should range somewhere between every one to four weeks, depending on their financial situation and the symptoms (emotional or physical) that the client is experiencing. For example, a client who is experiencing severe nausea or high levels of anxiety may be seen weekly, whereas a client who just wishes to receive reflexology for general wellbeing could be seen every 4 weeks.

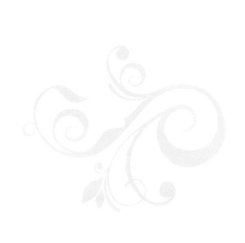

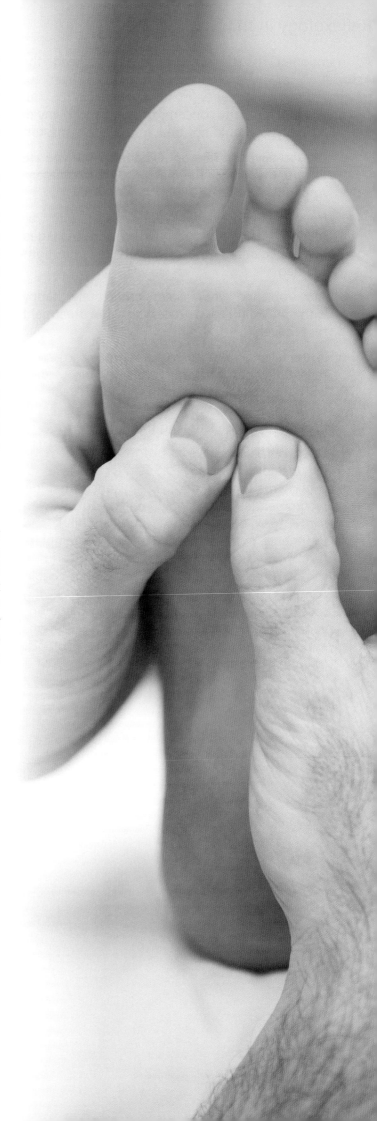

Treatment plan for the first trimester

Reflexology sequence

You can use your full sequence. Remember that your aim is to give a gentle, relaxing treatment to aid general well being, concentrating on reflexes for any symptoms that the client has at that time. Remember to use only light pressure on the uterus, ovaries, pituitary and thyroid (or avoid these areas if it feels right to you to do so).

N.B: remember:

1. If you use the 'ankle boogie' as an opening or closing move (where the palms of your hands move backwards and forwards behind the ankle bones), be careful not to apply pressure to the back of the heels (pelvic area) as this will add stimulation to the uterus and ovaries.

2. Do not work the chronic reproductive area (either side of leg) as this will pass over Spleen 6, which should not be worked (as discussed on page 106).

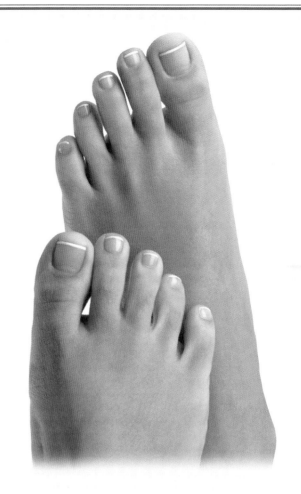

Reflex points to concentrate on for common symptoms

Morning sickness

Reflex point	Reason
Stomach – use unwind technique (p108)	Normalises stomach acid production
Pancreas and gall bladder	Regulates production of digestive enzymes
Thoracic spine	Normalises nerves to the area
Endocrine balance (p108-109)	Helps the client to adjust to changing hormones
Linking - gall bladder on itself - pinch on dorsal and plantar aspect of foot (see Appendix 2)	Eases tension within the digestive system

Fatigue or tiredness

Reflex point	Reason
Endocrine balance (p108-109)	Helps the client to adjust to changing hormones
Adrenal gland – if there has been long term stress	Aids the recovery of exhausted adrenals
Solar Plexus	Supports the client's life energy
Head, neck and shoulders	Alleviates feelings of heaviness

Breast tenderness

Reflex point	Reason
Breast area	Eases tension in the area
Thoracic spine	Normalises nerves to the area
Endocrine balance (p108-109)	Helps the client to adjust to changing hormones
Adrenal glands	Promotes the production of natural pain killers

Heartburn

Reflex point	Reason
Oesophagus	Helps to normalize function
Stomach, gall bladder and pancreas	Calms digestion
Adrenal glands	Promotes production of natural pain killers
Endocrine balance (p108-109)	Helps the client to adjust to changing hormones
Thoracic spine	Promotes nerve supply to the stomach and oesophagus
Linking – gall bladder to itself (see Appendix 2) and gentle circular movements over stomach area	Releases tension in the whole digestive system

Constipation

Reflex point	Reason
Large intestines	Encourages normal function
Small intestines	Assists digestion and absorption
Anus (if the client has haemorrhoids)	Relieves tension
Lumbar spine	Promotes nerve supply to the intestines
Linking - gall bladder on itself - pinch on dorsal and plantar aspect of foot (see Appendix 2)	Eases tension within the digestive system

Headaches

Reflex point	Reason
Head	Relieves tension in the area
Adrenal glands	Promotes production of natural pain killers
Cervical spine	Normalises nerves to the area
Endocrine balance (p108-109)	Helps the client to adjust to changing hormones
Linking – forebrain to sacrum (see Appendix 2)	Aids functioning of the central nervous system

Dizziness

Reflex point	Reason
Endocrine balance (p108-109)	Restores balance
Spine – use 'open spine technique' and spinal twist (p108)	Clears the central nervous system
Pancreas	Helps to regulate blood sugar levels
Liver and spleen	Supports red blood cell production
Linking – forebrain to sacrum (see Appendix 2)	Aids functioning of central nervous system

Anaemia

Reflex point	Reason
Spleen	Encourages red blood cell production
Liver	Normalises blood flow
Heart and cardiac area	Promotes circulation
Endocrine balance (p108-109)	Helps the client to adjust to changing hormones
Linking – adrenal reflex to groin reflex (see Appendix 2)	Promotes the circulatory system

Anxiety

Reflex point	Reason
Adrenal gland – unwind technique	Calms the production of adrenalin
Head, neck and shoulders	Releases tension
Solar plexus	Calms the client
Spine – use 'open spine technique' and spinal twist (p108)	Supports the central nervous system
Endocrine balance (p108-109)	Supports hormone balance
Linking – Lumbar 5 to hip (see Appendix 2)	Relaxes the nervous system

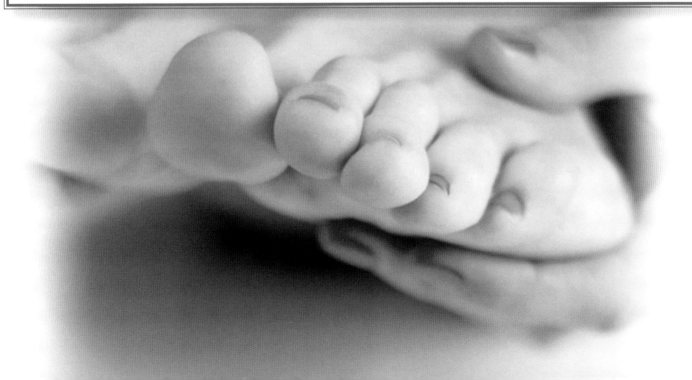

Common lifestyle advice for the second trimester

Increase in breast size

During the second trimester, the milk-producing glands inside the breasts get larger and additional fat may be laid down as a result of the increasing levels of oestrogen and progesterone. Although some of the initial breast tenderness is likely to improve, nipple tenderness might continue throughout the pregnancy. Once breasts begin to enlarge, a supportive bra that is not underwired should be worn.

Increase in libido

The high level of oestrogen boosts the blood flow to the pelvic region, making sexual arousal more frequent, and some women report heightened orgasms. It is perfectly safe to make love during pregnancy, although it does need to be gentle.

Constipation

This is a symptom that may occur throughout the pregnancy. The high level of progesterone causes the muscles of the intestines to slow and the pressure of the growing uterus will begin to push on the bowels, further inhibiting normal bowel movements. Mothers should be encouraged to drink plenty of water, eat foods rich in fibre and take regular exercise.

Changes in skin and hair

As blood circulation to the skin increases, certain areas of the skin often become darker, such as the areola (skin around the nipple), parts of the face and the line that runs from the navel down to the pubic bone. Stretch marks may appear as pink, red or purple streaks along the abdomen, breasts, upper arms, buttocks or thighs as the skin stretches - this may also cause itchiness. Encourage the woman to use an oil or cream to moisturise. The stretch marks should fade after the birth, although they may not disappear altogether.

Hair also appears thicker during pregnancy; higher levels of oestrogen prolong the growth phase of hair, resulting in less hair falling out on a daily basis. Some women also notice that their hair becomes shinier during pregnancy, or that it changes in texture. After the birth, the shedding of hair will resume and many women feel concerned about the amount of hair that appears to be falling out; however, they can be reassured that this is to be expected.

Sinus and gum changes.

During pregnancy, circulation increases and blood flow through mucous membranes increases. This causes the lining of the nose and airway to swell slightly, which in turn can restrict airflow and lead to snoring, congestion and nosebleeds. Some clients may find it beneficial to reduce dairy in their diet, but it is essential that they replace the dairy with other foods high in calcium e.g. sesame seeds, green leafy vegetables, soya and brazil nuts.

Increased blood circulation can also soften gums, which might cause minor bleeding when brushing or flossing teeth and can increase the risk of gum disease. Switching to a softer toothbrush can help and regular dental checks are essential.

At the time of publishing, NHS dental care is free for pregnant women and also for one year after the birth of their baby.

Dizziness

Blood vessels begin to dilate in response to pregnancy hormones and until the blood volume can increase to fill the larger capacity, blood pressure will fall temporarily, causing occasional bouts of dizziness. If a woman has trouble with dizziness, she should drink plenty of fluids and rise slowly after lying or sitting down, so this is especially important to consider at the end of a reflexology treatment. If a client feels dizzy, they should lie on their left side to restore blood pressure.

It is worth mentioning here about supine hypotension syndrome, which can be experienced by women in pregnancy. This usually occurs in the third trimester but can occasionally occur towards the end of the second trimester. It is characterized by a feeling of dizziness and nausea when a woman lies on her back. In very rare exceptions, it is possible for the pregnant woman to lose consciousness. It is caused by the pressure of the enlarged uterus and foetus pushing on (and partially obstructing), the inferior vena cava, which flows behind the uterus towards the heart. This compression of the vein can lead to decreased blood flow back to the heart, causing an eventual decrease in blood pressure and perfusion of the placenta.

Compression of this big vein usually occurs when the woman lies directly on her back, so as the pregnancy progresses it is important that during a treatment you either sit the client fairly upright, or if you are using a Lafuma chair, ask the woman to roll slightly onto her left side and place a cushion or wedge under her back to keep her in this position. Always ask your client to let you know if she experiences either breathlessness or dizziness at any time so you can correct her position.

Leg cramps

Leg cramps are also common as pregnancy progresses, often causing problems at night. To help prevent leg cramps during pregnancy, encourage the woman to stretch her calf muscles before going to bed. It also helps if she stays physically active and drinks plenty of fluids. If a leg cramp occurs during a treatment, stretch the calf muscle on the affected side; if this does not relieve it, she may have to stand up on tip toes. Pregnant women are at high risk of developing a deep vein thrombosis, so if cramp is not relieved by stretching, suspect DVT and seek emergency advice.

Braxton Hicks contractions

Towards the end of the second trimester and throughout the third trimester, the uterus might start contracting intermittently, practising for the birth ahead. These are called Braxton Hicks contractions, and are felt in the lower abdomen and groin. They're usually weak and come and go unpredictably. Your client should contact their midwife or doctor if her contractions become painful or regular.

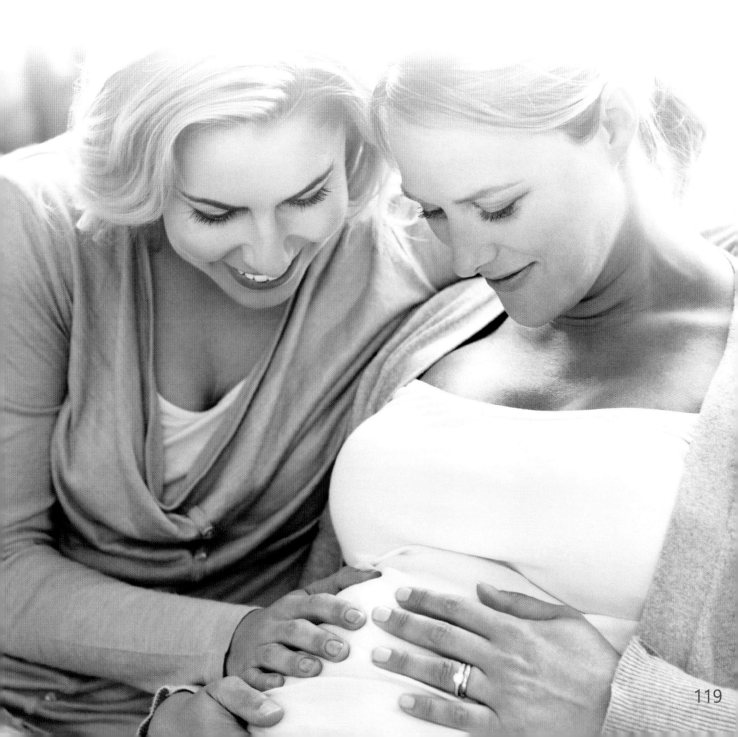

Reflexology in the second trimester

As stated, it is essential that you have read the Association of Reflexologists' information sheet in detail (pages 73-76), but certainly if you have any concerns or doubts with any of the following, you should not treat in the second trimester:

1. Have you provided your client with all relevant information, discussed and managed her expectations and answered any questions she had?

2. Both reflexologist and client must be completely happy with providing and receiving the treatment respectively.

3. Does the client have any contraindications? Refer to the Association of Reflexologists' information sheet (pages 73-76) and the standard Reflexology Forum contraindications list.

Are there any reflex points that should be avoided?

As with the first trimester, the only point thought to possibly cause problems in acupuncture is Spleen 6; this is discussed on page 106. Also be aware that if you work the chronic pelvic area by stimulating up either side of the ankle bone and calf muscle, you will in fact be working over Spleen 6, so this move should not be used until post 37 weeks.

Some schools teach that the ovaries, uterus, pituitary and thyroid should be avoided at all times throughout pregnancy. Current information suggests that there is no reason to avoid these reflexes, but neither is it recommended that you should specifically work into these areas.

Dos and don'ts

- Do focus on the client's health and any symptoms they may be experiencing.

- Do take extra care to ensure client comfort, especially towards the end of the second trimester when they will need to sit in a more upright position, or on their left side to avoid supine hypotension.

- Do allow extra time between ending the session and the client standing up.

- Do research and understand your subject.

- Do attend a CPD workshop/course on pregnancy.

- Don't exceed your training and experience.

- Don't treat pregnancy as an illness.

- Don't have the room too warm.

- Do be aware of smells in the treatment room - some pregnant women have a very sensitive sense of smell!

- Don't use or burn any essential oils unless you are qualified to do so throughout the client's pregnancy.

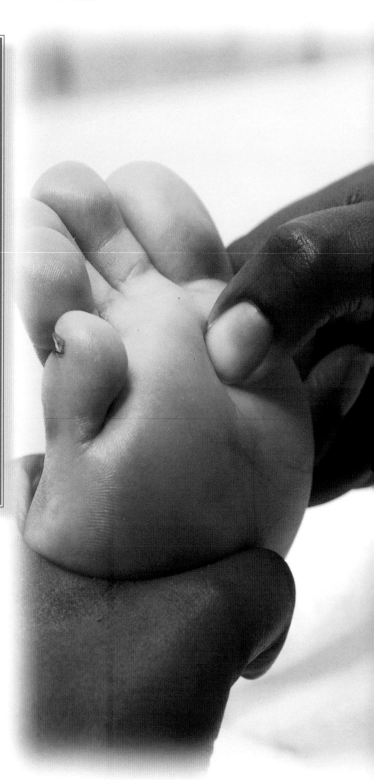

Treatment plan for the second trimester

You can use your full sequence in the second trimester, but remember that your aim is to aid general well being and promote relaxation. Spend time concentrating on reflex points for any symptoms the client has at that specific time. Some therapists still use only gentle pressure on the uterus, ovaries, pituitary and thyroid, and there is no evidence to say these should be avoided. Whilst they do not need extra time spent on them, generally they can be worked with normal/light pressure.

Receiving reflexology during pregnancy will also allow the woman time away from her probably busy life and a place where she should be able to focus purely on herself and her growing baby.

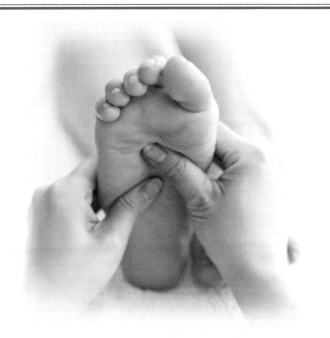

Reflex points to concentrate on for common symptoms

Constipation

Reflex point	Reason
Large intestines	Encourages normal function
Small intestines	Assists digestion and absorption
Anus (if the client has haemorrhoids)	Relieves tension
Lumbar spine	Promotes nerve supply to the intestines
Linking - gall bladder on itself - pinch on dorsal and plantar aspect of foot (see Appendix 2)	Eases tension within the digestive system

Sinus problems

Reflex point	Reason
Sinuses	Helps to normalise the production of mucous
Lungs	Helps to relieve any inflammation
Lymphatics	Aids detoxification of the area
Ileocaecal valve	Helps to normalise the production of mucous
Cervical spine	Promotes nerve supply to the sinuses
Linking – thymus to itself (dorsal and plantar - see Appendix 2)	Promotes the function of the lymphatic system

Bleeding gums

Reflex point	Reason
Jaw and teeth	Promotes healing
Lymphatics	Aids the removal of infection from the area
Cervical spine	Helps to regulate nerve supply to the area
Linking – thymus to itself (dorsal and plantar (see Appendix 2)	Promotes the function of the lymphatic system

Dizziness

Reflex point	Reason
Endocrine balance (p108-109)	Restores balance
Spine – use 'open spine technique' and spinal twist (p108)	Clears the central nervous system
Pancreas	Helps to regulate blood sugar levels
Liver and spleen	Supports red blood cell production
Linking – forebrain to sacrum (see Appendix 2)	Aids the functioning of the central nervous system

Common symptoms and lifestyle advice for the third trimester

Backache

Backache is experienced to some degree by up to three quarters of pregnant women. There are two main reasons for backache; firstly, as the baby continues to gain weight, muscles may get tired and ligaments stretch slightly from the additional weight. Secondly, pregnancy hormones relax the joints between the bones in your pelvic area and these two factors can put the body off balance, meaning that the back will have to work harder to maintain posture.

Advice for clients with backache

When they sit, they should choose chairs with good back support. They can try applying a heat pad or ice pack to the painful area or ask their partner for a massage. Footwear can also be a problem; by now, they should be wearing low-heeled - but not flat - shoes with good arch support. If the back pain doesn't go away or is accompanied by other signs and symptoms, they should contact their health care provider.

Breathlessness

Towards the end of the third trimester, the size of the growing baby can make the mother feel breathless. At this stage, the uterus really begins to push upwards into the mother's diaphragm, which reduces lung capacity, causing breathlessness. This is normal and harmless to mother and baby.

Breathlessness can also be a sign of anaemia. Check that your client is having regular full blood counts. Also, if the client is asthmatic, they should consult their doctor regarding management of their asthma as it can be worse during pregnancy.

Most women who are pregnant for the first time find that their baby drops down into their pelvis from about 36 weeks. This can help ease some of the breathlessness. If the mother has had a baby before, the baby might not drop down until the very end of the pregnancy.

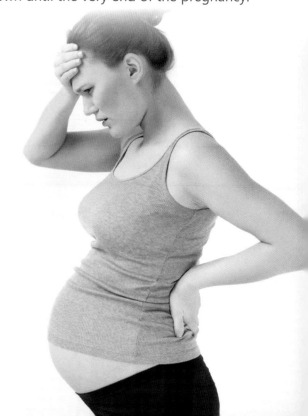

When is breathlessness a concern?

Some breathlessness is common and normal during pregnancy. However, your client needs to see a doctor or midwife immediately if they notice other worrying symptoms, such as:

- a feeling that their heart beat is racing, irregular or missing a beat.

- severe breathlessness or feeling faint after a burst of activity.

- chest pain, especially if it starts when they exert themselves.

Advice for breathlessness

Some light exercise generally helps. If the mother is unfit, they are more likely to feel breathless.

Gentle exercise means exercise that does not prevent the woman holding a conversation because they are short of breath e.g. walking, swimming, ante-natal yoga, ante-natal aqua aerobics.

Swollen ankles and hands

Between 50 per cent and 80 per cent of healthy pregnant women have oedema in the third trimester and hot weather can make it worse. This can be an issue as the body is holding onto excess fluid due to the extra blood circulating in the body. Also, as the uterus grows it puts pressure on the veins (particularly the inferior vena cava), which means that venous return is slowed down. Pressure from this excess of blood in the extremities forces water down and out through the capillaries and into the tissues of feet, ankles and hands. Swelling in legs, arms or hands can also place pressure on nerves, causing tingling or numbness.

There is often less swelling in the morning after the woman has been lying in bed; as the day goes on, more swelling appears. Later in the day, the oedema may become noticeable and the woman will experience tightness of the skin. Towards the end of the pregnancy, the swelling may affect hands, making rings feel tight on fingers.

If the woman experiences sudden or severe swelling in their face, hands or feet, they should call their doctor or midwife as it could be a sign of pre-eclampsia, which can be a serious condition for both mother and baby.

Advice for oedema

- They should elevate their feet when sitting to help venous return. At work, they should try and put feet up onto a footstool under their desk and at home, they should try to lie down on their left side to take pressure off the inferior vena cava.

- They should put on support tights before they get out of bed in the morning, so blood has no chance to pool around the ankles.

- They should drink plenty of water. Surprisingly, keeping hydrated helps the body to hoard less water.

- They should take regular gentle exercise, especially walking, swimming or gentle cycling, which can encourage venous return.

- If they are travelling long distances, they should take regular breaks to stretch their legs.

- They should eat well, avoiding high-sodium and salty foods, such as olives and salted nuts.

- Gentle upward massage of ankles and feet (towards the knees) can help to move the fluid away from their feet.

Pre-eclampsia

This affects approximately 10% of women. It can occur from as early as 20 weeks, or as late as after the birth, but it is more likely after 27 weeks. It can be potentially harmful to both the mother and the baby, causing growth problems for the foetus. In some cases, further complications can develop, such as eclampsia. This is a type of seizure that can be life-threatening for the mother and the baby. However, this is rare and less than 1% of women with pre-eclampsia develop eclampsia.

Complications resulting from pre-eclampsia are responsible for the deaths of around six women every year in the UK. Several hundred babies also die each year following complications from severe pre-eclampsia, often as a result of premature birth. Therefore, the earlier that pre-eclampsia is diagnosed and monitored, the better the outlook for mother and baby.

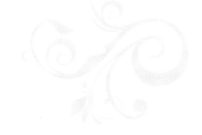

Pregnant women with pre-eclampsia may not realise they have it. Pre-eclampsia is usually diagnosed during routine ante-natal appointments. Symptoms include:

- hypertension.
- proteinuria (protein in the urine).

They probably won't notice these symptoms, but their GP or midwife should pick them up during ante-natal appointments.

Other signs that they may experience are:

- severe oedema which often causes sudden swelling of the feet, ankles, face and hands.
- severe headaches.
- vision problems, such as blurring or seeing flashing lights.
- pain in the epigastrum (the part of the upper abdomen immediately over the stomach)
- vomiting.
- excessive weight gain due to fluid retention.
- feeling generally unwell.

If they notice any symptoms of pre-eclampsia, they should seek medical advice immediately.

Without immediate treatment, pre-eclampsia may lead to a number of serious complications, including:

- eclampsia (convulsions).
- HELLP syndrome - a combined liver and blood clotting disorder.
- stroke.

Symptoms in the unborn baby

The main sign of pre-eclampsia in the unborn baby is slow growth, which should be picked up on routine scans. This is caused by poor blood supply through the placenta to the baby.

The growing baby receives less oxygen and fewer nutrients than it should, which can affect development. This is called intra-uterine growth restriction, or intra-uterine growth retardation.

Dizziness

See the information presented for the second trimester, but remember about supine hypotension syndrome, which usually occurs in the third trimester. It is characterised by a feeling of dizziness and nausea when a woman lies on her back. In very rare exceptions it is possible for the pregnant woman to lose consciousness. It is caused by the pressure of the enlarged uterus and the baby pushing on (and partially obstructing), the inferior vena cava, which flows behind the uterus towards the heart. This compression of the vein can lead to decreased blood flow back to the heart, and eventual decrease in blood pressure.

Remember: when treating clients in the third trimester, keep them upright and tilted onto their left side. If they begin to feel breathless or faint, get them to lie over onto their left side.

Heartburn

Many women experience heartburn in the third trimester; this should not cause any harm, but can be painful. Heartburn is a burning sensation that often extends down from the lower throat. It happens when stomach acid is brought up into the oesophagus. The acid may come up into the throat or mouth, leaving a sour and bitter taste.

It is thought to be caused by both hormonal and physical changes in the body. An increase in the hormone progesterone in pregnancy relaxes the smooth muscles of the uterus. However, this also relaxes the oesophageal sphincter, which allows gastric acid to seep back up the oesophagus. This causes a burning sensation. Progesterone also slows down the peristalsis in the stomach, making digestion sluggish. In later pregnancy, the growing foetus also pushes the intestines and stomach upwards. This slows digestion and forces acids up from the stomach into the oesophagus. These symptoms will disappear once the baby drops down into the pelvis or after birth.

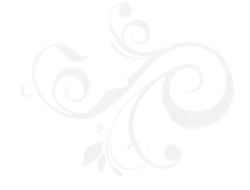

Advice for clients with heartburn

The main triggers are eating, lying down and bending over. Ask your client to try and work out which activities make heartburn worse for them, so they can try to avoid them. Although it is hard to eliminate heartburn entirely, some of the following may give your client some relief:

- Choosing foods and drinks that are easy to digest. She should avoid rich, high-fat or spicy dishes, chocolate, citrus fruits or juices, alcohol and coffee.

- A milky drink can help to settle heartburn. It is generally better to choose semi skimmed or skimmed milk as these are lower in fat.

- Eating small, frequent meals regularly. This leaves less time for acid to build up in the client's stomach as food neutralises stomach acid.

- If the client is still smoking, this will also make heartburn worse, as well as the other risks already discussed. Smoking further relaxes the oesophageal sphyncter, making acid reflux more likely to happen.

- Keep the client upright, particularly during and just after meals. She should sit up straight and try not to bend over or slump. Wearing loose clothes around the stomach may help, and she should try not to lie down for at least an hour after eating.

- If heartburn is worse at night, the client should try not to eat or drink anything but water for the three hours before she goes to bed.

- Sleeping in a propped-up position. Suggest that your client uses several pillows, or raises the head of the bed with some cushions. Gravity will help to keep her stomach acids in her stomach.

- If she is on any medication, she should consult her doctor or midwife to check these are not adding to the indigestion e.g. antidepressants and non-steroidal anti-inflammatory drugs aggravate indigestion and there may be alternatives.

- Some over-the-counter antacids may give relief; this should be discussed with the doctor, midwife or pharmacist to ensure that the medicine is safe in pregnancy.

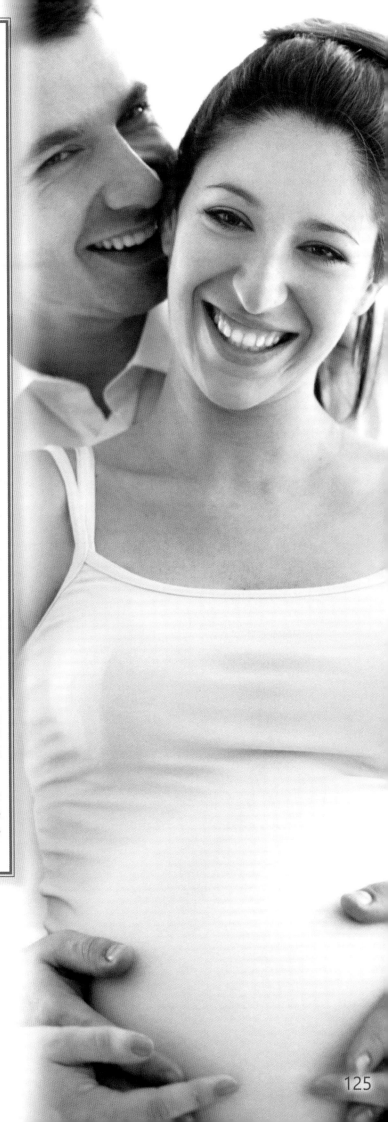

Gestational diabetes

Gestational diabetes is a type of diabetes that affects about 10% of pregnant women. Normally, the amount of glucose in the blood is controlled by the hormone insulin. However, during pregnancy, some women have slightly higher than normal levels of glucose in their blood and either their body cannot produce enough insulin or their body develops insulin resistance. This means that the level of glucose in the blood rises.

Gestational diabetes can usually be controlled with diet and exercise. Approximately 15% of women with gestational diabetes will require medication to control their blood glucose levels.

Gestational diabetes is usually picked up by routine blood tests taken during ante-natal appointments before it causes any problems. If it goes undiagnosed, the woman may experience:

- Thirst
- Dry mouth
- Frequent urination
- Tiredness
- Recurrent infections, such as thrush
- Blurred vision

If gestational diabetes goes undetected or is not managed effectively, it can cause complications for both the mother and baby.

Undiagnosed or poorly managed gestational diabetes may increase the risk of:

- Pre-eclampsia
- Placental abruption (the placenta starts to come away from the wall of the uterus)
- Premature birth
- Macrosomia (baby is larger than average due to excess blood sugar levels)
- Trauma during the birth due to the macrosomia
- Neonatal hypoglycaemia (the newborn baby may have low blood glucose), which can cause poor feeding, blue-tinged skin and irritability
- Perinatal death (the death of the baby around the time of the birth)

Future implications

After having gestational diabetes, a woman is more likely to develop type 2 diabetes than women who have had a normal pregnancy.

There is an increased risk of having gestational diabetes in any future pregnancies.

The baby may also be at greater risk of developing diabetes or obesity in later life.

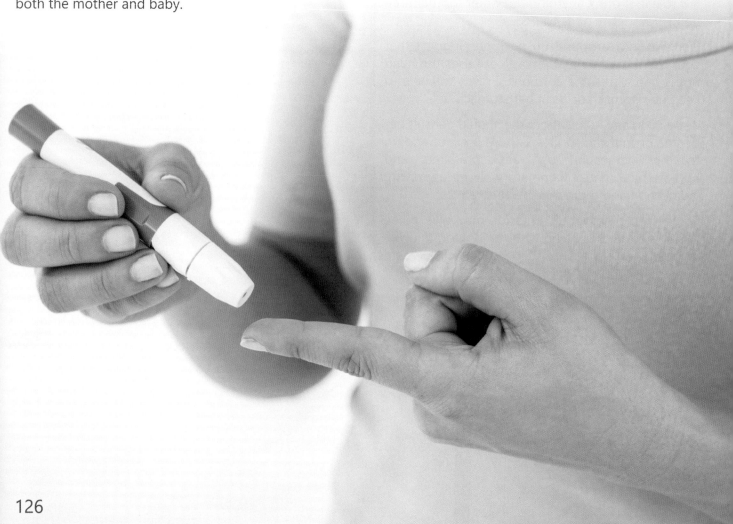

Haemorrhoids

Haemorrhoids are blood vessels in the rectal area that have become unusually swollen. They typically range from the size of a pea to the size of a grape and can be inside the rectum or protruding through the anus. They can be itchy, mildly uncomfortable or very painful. They can even cause rectal bleeding, especially during a bowel movement.

Haemorrhoids are common during pregnancy, particularly in the third trimester. Some women get them for the first time whilst they are pregnant. If they have had them before pregnancy, then they are more likely to have them during pregnancy. They may also develop during the second stage of labour and are a common early post-natal complaint. In most cases, haemorrhoids that developed during pregnancy will begin to resolve soon after birth, but it is important that the woman tries to avoid becoming constipated.

Pregnancy makes women more prone to haemorrhoids, as well as to varicose veins in the legs for a variety of reasons:

- The growing uterus puts pressure on the pelvic veins and the inferior vena cava: this can slow the return of blood from the lower half of the body, which increases the pressure on the veins below the uterus and causes them to become more dilated or swollen.

- Constipation is another common problem during pregnancy: this can also cause or aggravate haemorrhoids.

- The increase in the hormone progesterone during pregnancy causes the walls of the veins to relax, allowing them to swell more easily. Progesterone also contributes to constipation by slowing down the intestinal tract.

Advice for clients with haemorrhoids

- They should avoid constipation by eating a high-fibre diet (plenty of whole grains, beans, fruits, and vegetables). Drinking plenty of water and getting regular exercise may be helpful too.

- If they are constipated, they could speak to their doctor, midwife or pharmacist about using a fibre supplement, stool softener or haemorrhoid treatments.

- They should try not to strain when moving their bowels and they should not sit for too long on the toilet, as this puts pressure on the area.

- They should avoid sitting or standing for long stretches of time. If their job involves a lot of sitting, they need to get up and move around for a few minutes every hour. At home, they can lie on their left side when sleeping, reading, or watching TV to take the pressure off the rectal veins and help increase blood return from the lower half of the body.

- They could apply a covered ice pack to the affected area several times a day. Ice may help decrease swelling and discomfort.

- They could try alternating cold and warm treatments. An ice pack followed by a warm bath can bring relief.

- The anus should be thoroughly cleaned after each bowel movement using soft, unscented, white toilet tissue, which causes less irritation than coloured, scented varieties. Some women find it more comfortable to use moistened wipes.

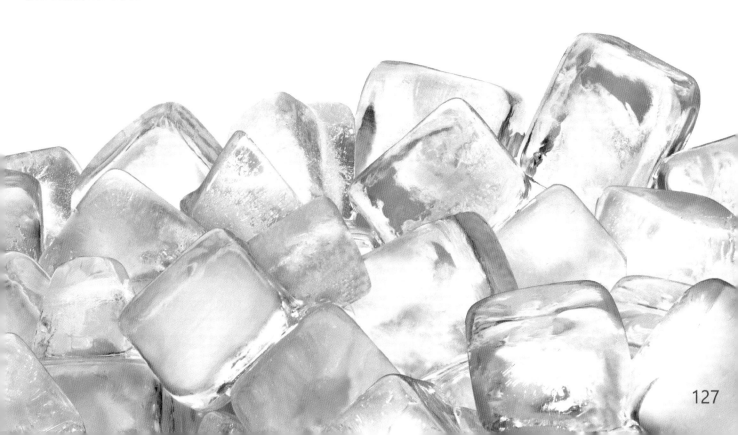

Varicose veins

Varicose veins present as bulging purple or blue veins, showing generally on calves. Although veins do not have muscular walls to pump blood back to the heart, they do have valves that stop the blood from flowing backwards. Varicose veins develop when the valves don't work properly and the vein walls become weak. Blood collects in the area of weakness. Once this has happened, the walls of the vein start to stretch and sag, the vein itself swells and can then be seen under the skin.

The reason that varicose veins are common in pregnancy is for similar reasons to haemorrhoids. The growing uterus puts pressure on the veins in the pelvis including the inferior vena cava, making venous return harder. Progesterone relaxes the blood vessel walls, meaning the veins are more likely to become swollen or varicose. They do generally improve after the birth.

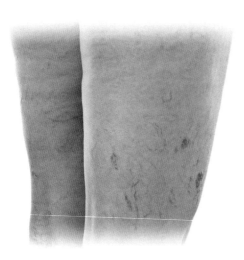

Advice for clients with varicose veins

- They should lie down or sleep on their left side to take the pressure off the inferior vena cava.

- They shouldn't sit or stand for long periods of time. Instead, they should move around at least once every half an hour. Gentle exercise will help improve circulation. Even a quick, brisk walk can help.

- They should not cross their legs. Instead, they should put their feet up whenever they can. To do this, they could use a footstool or box.

- If they put on too much weight, too quickly, it may make them more prone to varicose veins. Instead, they should try to follow a healthy, balanced diet.

- There are various tights and stockings that can help, from maternity support tights to compression stockings which their doctor can prescribe.

- Tights or stockings must be put on before they get out of bed in the morning to prevent blood pooling in the lower leg. There is no guarantee that tights or stockings will stop varicose veins from getting worse, but they may help control swelling and discomfort.

Frequent urination

Both the frequency of urination (micturition) and volume of urine generally increase over the course of the pregnancy. Shortly after women become pregnant, hormonal changes cause blood to flow more quickly through the kidneys, filling the bladder more often. As blood volume increases, this leads to a lot of extra fluid being processed through the kidneys.

As pregnancy progresses and the baby moves lower into the pelvis, this will put more pressure on the bladder, which can lead to needing to urinate more often - even during the night. This extra pressure might also cause mild incontinence, especially when they laugh, cough or sneeze. Additionally, they need to watch for signs of a urinary tract infection, such as urinating even more than usual, burning during urination, fever, abdominal pain or backache. Left untreated, urinary infections increase the risk of pregnancy complications.

Advice for clients experiencing more frequent urination

- They should avoid beverages that have a mild diuretic effect, such as coffee, tea and alcohol (they should not be really be drinking any of these anyway!)

- They should wear panty liners or small incontinence pads, which are now widely available in chemists.

- When they pass urine, they should lean forward to help completely empty the bladder.

- They should not reduce the amount of water they drink. This can change the pH balance of the urine, which irritates the bladder and can lead to the feeling of needing to urinate even more. Also, it is important for the health of the mother and baby that they stay well hydrated.

- They can try drinking plenty of fluids during the day but then cutting back before bed.

Braxton Hicks

Towards the end of the second trimester and throughout the third trimester, the uterus might start contracting intermittently, practising for the birth ahead. Braxton Hicks are felt in the lower abdomen and groin. These become more frequent and stronger as the pregnancy progresses but will not last for long. If these become painful and regular they should contact their midwife or doctor.

Fatigue

Tiredness is common in the first trimester and then tends to disappear in the second trimester. However, it can return as the growing foetus puts more demands on the body and anxiety about the birth may cause disturbed nights. Also, sleep can often be disturbed because the woman finds it hard to get comfortable and may need to visit the loo several times in the night. Some people say it is the woman's way of preparing for the months of sleepless nights that are to come – but this is not very helpful information for an exhausted woman!

Advice for clients experiencing fatigue

- They should listen to the body's signals by taking catnaps or going to bed early. Even a 20-minute nap can make a difference.

- They should adjust their schedule: if possible, they should try to arrange to work from home occasionally or, if they are at home with other children, they should try and have a break now and then to leave their children with someone else in order to have a nap.

- They should eat properly - A healthy diet made up of vegetables, fruits, wholegrains, skimmed milk and lean meats can be energising; junk food actually saps energy levels. Eating and drinking little and often may help with nausea and vomiting.

- They need to hang in there – it will not be long until they are holding their baby, which will make it all worthwhile.

Anxiety

The third trimester is the time which is full of anticipation. Soon, the nine months will come to an end and the baby will at last be born. First-time mothers may have especially high levels of anxiety with fear about childbirth. They may be worrying about pain in labour, how long it will last and if they will be able to manage through the delivery. They may even start to be concerned about how they will manage with looking after a newborn, breastfeeding, lack of sleep, etc.

For those who know they will have to have a caesarian section, there are fears associated with the surgery itself, as well as common post operative complications such as pain management and recovery time, including not being able to drive for up to 6 weeks.

These fears and thoughts are completely normal, so spend time allowing clients to talk through their worries and concerns; reassure them these feelings are completely normal. It may also be worth reminding them that however the baby is born, at least they will be able to hold and cuddle him/her very soon. If anxiety levels seem excessive, recommend that your client discusses this with her midwife or doctor; they are there to support both with physical and emotional troubles.

Advice for clients experiencing anxiety

Pregnant women should be offered NHS ante-natal classes; these are invaluable to help educate 'parents to be' on what to expect, common childbirth issues, and to offer reassurance on common concerns. They will also provide an opportunity to have any questions answered.

If your client can afford to pay for additional classes, the National Childbirth Trust (www.nct.org.uk) also offer excellent ante-natal classes.

All classes will be local and will also let your client meet other local pregnant woman who will love to share stories about pregnancy and hopefully reflexology! These may even become good friends to her, who she will meet up with after the births of their babies.

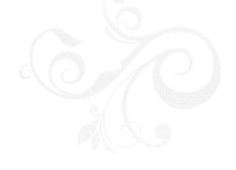

Depression

Most people have heard of post-natal depression, but it is estimated that up to 1 in 10 women will suffer from some depression during their pregnancy. It is thought that the increase in hormones can change brain chemistry and leave some women prone to depression. The number of women experiencing depression may actually be more than 10%, because it is believed that many women just put it down to 'hormonal moodiness'. However, seeking help for depression is worthwhile. Also, those who have depression during their pregnancy are at higher risk of post-natal depression, so they must be carefully monitored.

The symptoms of depression are described at www.nhs.uk/Conditions/Depression. These can be complex and vary widely between people. But as a general rule, if they are depressed, feel sad, hopeless and lose interest in things they used to enjoy – and if these symptoms persist for weeks or months, being bad enough to interfere with their work, social life and family life, then they should seek help.

Psychological symptoms include:

- continuous low mood or sadness
- feeling hopeless and helpless
- having low self-esteem
- feeling tearful
- feeling guilt-ridden
- feeling irritable and intolerant of others
- having no motivation or interest in things
- finding it difficult to make decisions
- not getting any enjoyment out of life
- having suicidal thoughts or thoughts of harming themselves
- feeling anxious or worried
- moving or speaking more slowly than usual
- changes in appetite or weight (usually decreased, but sometimes increased)
- constipation
- unexplained aches and pains
- lack of energy or lack of interest in sex
- disturbed sleep (for example, finding it hard to fall asleep at night or waking up very early in the morning)

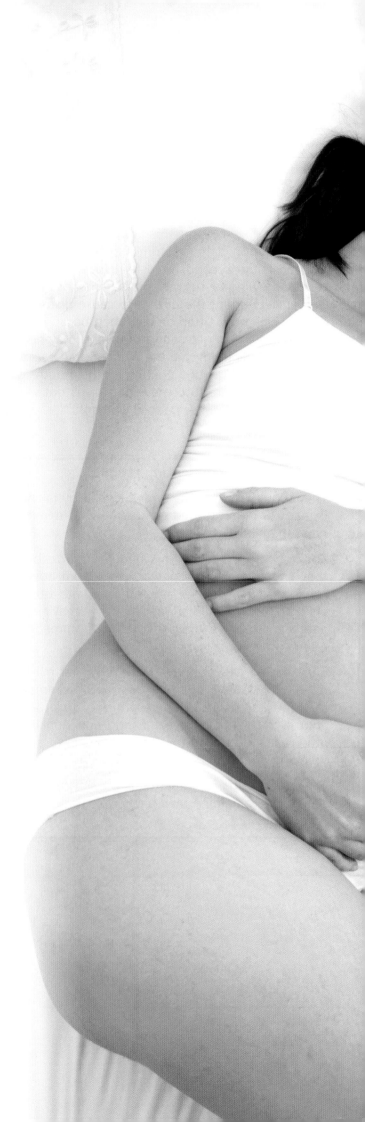

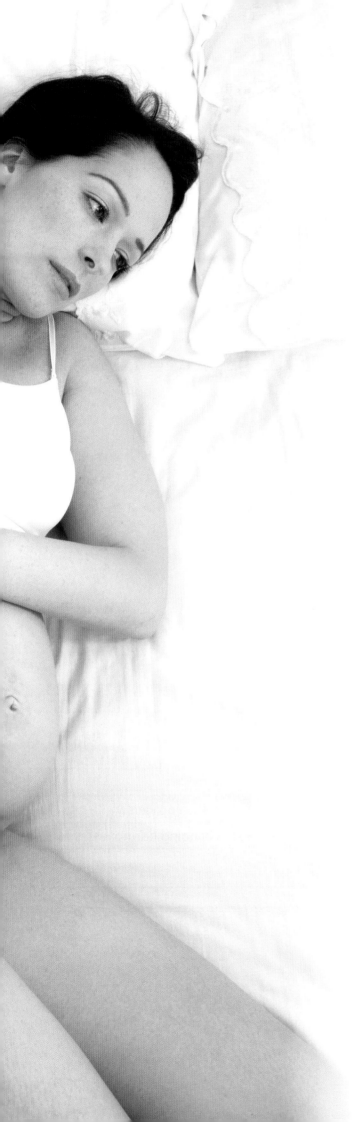

Social symptoms include:

- not doing well at work

- taking part in fewer social activities and avoiding contact with friends

- neglecting hobbies and interests

- having difficulties in home and family life

If they experience some of these symptoms for most of the day, every day for more than two weeks, they should seek help from their GP. There a few lifestyle factors that can help raise mood which are listed below, but you must encourage your client to seek medical help if you fear they may be depressed.

Advice for clients experiencing depression

- They should be active by taking up some form of exercise. There's evidence that exercise can help lift the mood. They could start gently by walking for 20 minutes every day.

- They should socialise: The client shouldn't withdraw from life. Socializing can improve mood and keeping in touch with friends and family means they have someone to talk to when they feel low.

- They need to face their fears: they should not avoid the things they find difficult. When people feel low or anxious, they sometimes avoid talking to other people. Some people can lose their confidence e.g. about driving or travelling. If this starts to happen, facing up to these situations will help them become easier.

- They must not turn to alcohol: this is not only bad for the baby; although alcohol can make people feel better in the short term because it raises opioid levels, it does not help deal with the depression in the longer term and can make it worse.

- They should have a sleep routine: when people feel low they can get into poor sleep patterns by staying up late and sleeping during the day. They should try to get up at their normal time and stick to a routine as much as possible.

- They should eat well: eating can be affected by depression (either they might not be eating, or they might be comfort eating - particularly on poor nutritional snacks such as chocolate and crisps).

Reflexology in the third trimester

This has been split into two sections, mainly because up until week 37, your treatment will remain the same in principle as for the second trimester. However, there may be extra symptoms that will require you to spend longer on certain reflexes. After 37 weeks, your treatment will change as you alter the treatment to prepare for labour.

Weeks 28-37

This remains exactly the same as for the second trimester, so please refer back to pages 121-122.

Reflexology sequence

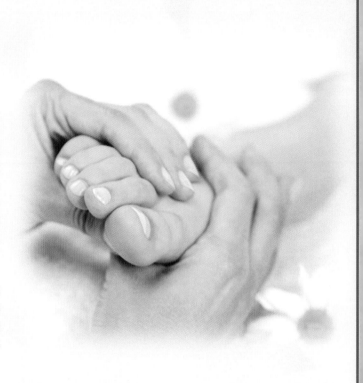

You can use your full sequence in weeks 28 - 37 but remember: your aim is to aid general wellbeing and promote relaxation. Spend time concentrating on reflex points for any symptoms the client has at that specific time. Some therapists still use only gentle pressure on the uterus, ovaries, pituitary and thyroid, but there is no evidence to say these should be avoided. Whilst they do not need extra time spent on them, generally they can be worked with normal/light pressure.

As this is the time when anxieties tend to arise, it is important that you spend time listening to your client's worries, reassuring her or suggesting she discusses these with her midwife or doctor if you are concerned about what she is expressing.

Reflex points to concentrate on for common symptoms

Please refer back again to the second trimester for those symptoms that may have started in second trimester. Below are extra symptoms that may be new in third trimester.

Backache

Reflex point	Reason
Work the spine reflexes several times; try using small circular moves along the spine on one of your walks.	Eases tension
Sciatic loop	Relieves pressure
Adrenal glands	Promotes production of natural pain killers
Endocrine balance (p108-109)	Helps the client to adjust to changing hormones
Linking – Lumbar 5 to hip (see Appendix 2)	Relaxes the area

Breathlessness

Reflex point	Reason
Lungs and diaphragm line	Optimises function
Chest area	Relaxes the area
Endocrine balance (p108-109)	Helps the client to adjust to changing hormones
Thoracic spine	Promotes nerve supply to the lungs
Linking – any tender lung areas linked to spine (see Appendix 2)	Releases tension

Oedema

Reflex point	Reason
Plenty of gentle massage moves up the legs, stroking up towards the heart. Take it at least up to the popliteal node (knee height)	Encourages venous return and lymphatic drainage.
Gentle flexion of toes and ankle rotations	Promotes movement of lymph up the leg
Lymphatics of the groin and chest	Helps to normalise the lymphatic system
Endocrine balance (p108-109)	Helps the client to adjust to changing hormones
Lumbar spine	Promotes nerve supply to the legs
Linking – any tender lung areas linked to spine (see Appendix 2)	Releases tension

Heartburn

Reflex point	Reason
Oesophagus	Helps to normalise function
Stomach, gall bladder and pancreas	Calms digestion
Adrenal glands	Promotes production of natural pain killers
Endocrine balance (p108-109)	Helps the client to adjust to changing hormones
Thoracic spine	Promotes nerve supply to the stomach and oesophagus
Linking – gall bladder to itself (see Appendix 2) and gentle circular movements over stomach area	Releases tension in the whole digestive system

Haemorrhoids

Reflex point	Reason
Small and large intestines	Promotes normal bowel movements
Rectum / anus	Eases tension in the area
Heart and chest area	Eases pressure on the circulatory system
Adrenal glands	Promotes production of natural pain killers
Lumbar spine	Promotes nerve supply to the rectum/anus
Endocrine balance (p108-109)	Helps the client to adjust to changing hormones
Linking – gall bladder to itself (see Appendix 2) and gentle circular movements over stomach area	Releases tension in the whole digestive system

Varicose veins

Reflex point	Reason
Extremely gentle massage moves up the legs, stroking up towards the heart. No direct pressure or heat should be applied to obvious varicose veins	Encourages venous return.
Heart and chest area	Eases pressure on the circulatory system
Adrenal glands (if they cause pain)	Helps to normalise the lymphatic system
Lumbar spine	Promotes nerve supply to the legs
Endocrine balance (p108-109)	Helps the client to adjust to changing hormones
Linking – adrenal reflex to groin reflex (see Appendix 2)	Helps the client's circulatory system to adjust to increased blood volume

Frequent urination

Reflex point	Reason
Bladder	Eases tension
Kidney	Helps to normalise function
Massage pelvic area	Relaxes the pelvic area
Thoracic 12 – Lumbar 3	Promotes nerve supply to the kidneys
Lumbar spine and sacrum	Promotes nerve supply to the bladder
Endocrine balance (p108-109)	Helps the client to adjust to changing hormones
Linking – adrenal reflex to groin reflex (see Appendix 2)	Helps the circulatory system adjust to increased blood volume

Fatigue or tiredness

Reflex point	Reason
Endocrine balance (p108-109)	Promotes normal bowel movements
Adrenal gland – if there has been long term stress	Eases tension in the area
Solar Plexus	Eases pressure on the circulatory system
Head, neck and shoulders	Promotes production of natural pain killers

Anxiety

Reflex point	Reason
Adrenal gland – unwind technique	Calms the production of adrenalin
Head, neck and shoulders	Eases tension
Solar plexus	Calms the client
Spine – use 'open spine technique' and spinal twist (p108)	Supports the client's central nervous system
Endocrine balance (p108-109)	Supports hormone balance
Linking – Lumbar 5 to hip (see Appendix 2)	Relaxes the nervous system

Depression

Reflex point	Reason
Head and brain	Calms any chemical imbalances
Pituitary and hypothalamus	Helps to regulate hormones
Solar plexus	Calms nerves
Spine – use 'open spine technique' and spinal twist (p108)	Promotes the function of the nervous system
Endocrine balance (p108-109)	Supports hormone balance
Linking – Lumbar 5 to hip (see Appendix 2)	Relaxes the nervous system

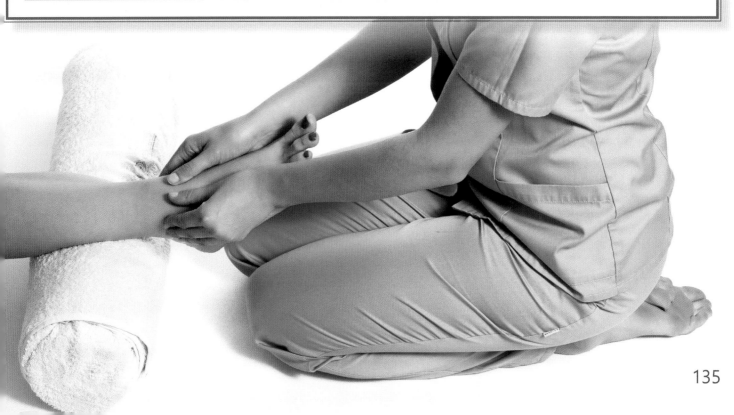

Breech baby

By week 36, the majority of babies will now be head down, but 3-4% will present in the breech position (bottom or legs facing the cervix). It is fairly common practice that if the baby is a breech presentation, a doctor may attempt to manually turn the baby by external manipulation (external cephalic version) around 37 weeks. The woman will have a scan to check if it would be safe to turn the baby (checking the position of the cord and the placenta). Once they have had their scan and the doctor has confirmed that it would be safe for the baby to turn, you could try to encourage them to have reflexology to see if this may help the baby to turn before the doctor tries to manually turn the baby (which can be very uncomfortable and some find it emotionally traumatic).

Although there is no evidence that reflexology can help a breech baby turn, I have seen babies turn on two occasions after receiving a treatment based on Traditional Chinese Medicine. This is a treatment based on stimulation using firm pressure and can be very strong. Therefore, it should not be undertaken lightly without training to understand fully when it can be used appropriately. Until you are have undertaken specialised training, try the following:

- Spend extra time working the uterus, coccyx and lumbar spine reflexes, and revisit these throughout your treatment.

- Use plenty of massage moves with your knuckles on the pelvic area to relax the area.

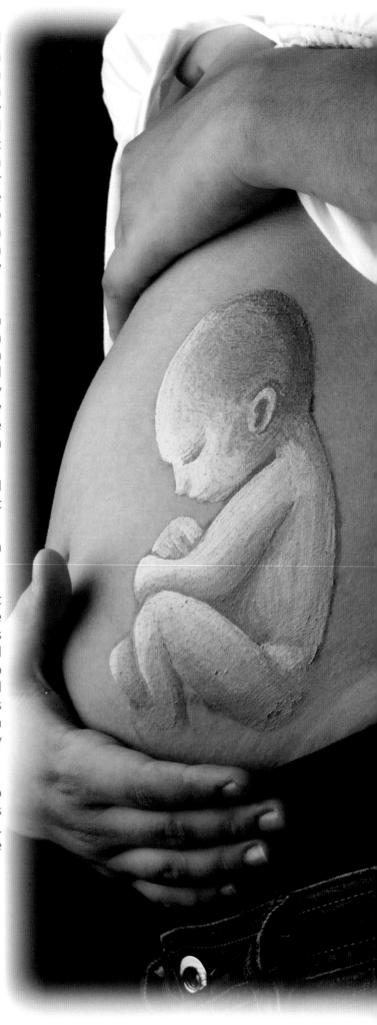

You may wish to suggest that she visits an acupuncturist who will use Moxa Sticks over specific acupressure points for turning a breech baby. Moxibustion involves the burning of a traditional Chinese herb stick and placing it near acupressure points. One end of the herb is lit so it smokes with a glowing ember. It is believed that the heat and herbs amplify the treatment. There is no evidence backing this as a treatment for turning a breech baby, but there are many women who swear by it.

After the reflexology treatment, advise your client to return home and try and spend some time on all fours – maybe over a bean bag if she finds it uncomfortable. This again allows extra space in the abdomen to give the baby more of a chance to turn.

Weeks 37+

Although there is no evidence that reflexology can induce labour, the general view is that it will help to support the body to prepare for labour and promote relaxation at a time when anxiety levels are often high.

The mechanisms regulating the onset of labour have remained obscure, but it can be helpful to know about three of the main hormones involved with reproduction: oxytocin, endorphins, and adrenaline. These hormones play a major role in regulating the process of labour and birth.

Oxytocin: This is produced by the pituitary gland and stimulates powerful contractions, which help to dilate the cervix.

Endorphins: These are produced by the pituitary gland and hypothalamus. In response to stress and pain, the body produces calming and pain-relieving hormones called endorphins. The level of this natural opiate may rise toward the end of pregnancy. High endorphin levels during labour and birth can produce an altered state of consciousness that can help women through the process, even if it is long and challenging.

Adrenalin: This is produced by the adrenal gland and is the "fight or flight" hormone that humans produce to help ensure survival. Women who feel threatened during labour (for example by fear or severe pain) may produce high levels of adrenalin. Adrenalin can slow labour or stop it altogether. Earlier in human evolution, it is believed that this slowing of labour helped birthing women move to a place of greater safety.

Reflexology to help prepare for labour

This is the time when you can start to increase your pressure and direct your treatment to help the body in preparing for labour. You may find that women will call and say they are 38, 39, 40 or even 41 weeks pregnant and have had no reflexology during their pregnancy. If this is the case, it is important that they receive two normal reflexology treatments before you increase the pressure, or else they are likely to experience a severe healing reaction.

Assuming they have been having regular reflexology, or have had their two 'normal' treatments, this is a time when you can see your women once or twice a week. On page 107, I talked about working the toe triangle, which ensures that the pituitary, hypothalamus and pineal are covered from all foot maps that I have come across. If you are unclear about the toe triangle, please refer back to page 107.

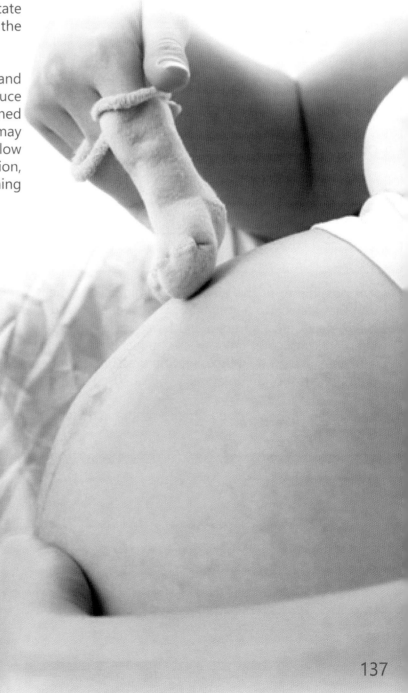

Preparing for labour

This is a treatment based on stimulation, using firm pressure on the areas outlined below and normal pressure on the rest of the reflexes. Try to revisit each of these points or areas 4-6 times in the treatment:

Reflex points to concentrate on

Reflex point	Reason
Toe triangle	Helps to prepare the pituitary and hypothalamus for increased production of oxytocin and endorphins.
Uterus	Helps to prepare the uterine wall ready for contractions.
Cervix/vagina  Both feet, from uterus point	Helps to prepare the cervix for the changes that are about to happen.
Pelvic area – use knuckles over this area	Eases tension in the area.
Adrenal glands	Helps to normalise the production of adrenalin. If stress levels are high, you can use the unwind technique over the reflex.
Lumbar spine, sacrum and coccyx	Relaxes the area.

Other useful techniques that can be used once during the treatment:

Reflex point	Reason
Endocrine balance (p108-109)	Supports hormone balance.
Linking – Forebrain to sacrum (see Appendix 2)	Helps to combat stress.

It is possible to fit this all into a 45 minute treatment. You can do your normal routine but spend less time on other areas. Do a little bit of your sequence and then break off and do your 'repeats'- toe triangle, uterus, cervix, pelvic area, adrenals and lower back – then return to where you were on your sequence and continue. Keep breaking off at times when you feel it is appropriate and do your repeats again until you have done them 4-6 times. You should be using firm pressure on your repeats – but stay within the comfort zone of your client; during the rest of the treatment, you can use your normal pressure.

Before you close is a good time to do the endocrine balance and linking, as these are a lovely, calming way to end.

Reflexology during labour

Before I talk about reflexology during labour, there are some things that need to be considered and some boundaries that need to be set. These should be discussed during the pregnancy so all is clear as to what each of you expect and are prepared to accept. As with setting any boundaries, there are no right or wrong answers - but it is down to you to decide:

- Do you have permission to attend the birth? The hospital or the midwife must be informed prior to the labour that you would like to attend, that you are only there to support the woman and that you will not offer any obstetric advice. They must agree, preferably in writing, that you are able to be present at the birth.

- Cost: what are you going to charge the client?

    - if you charge them a fixed fee then you may get a very low rate of pay or, if the birth is rapid, they may end up paying a very high rate.

    - If you charge an hourly rate, it could end up costing your client a small fortune.

    - If they have been a regular client, you might consider not charging if you feel you would like the experience of treating in labour.

- Times: are you willing to be called any time of night or day? How long are you prepared to be there for? You may have commitments of your own. Reflexology is most likely to be used during first stage, so discuss with your client what you can offer to ensure these match her expectations.

- Your role: make it clear you are only there as a support for the woman. The midwife or doctor is solely responsible for guidance on the birth, and remains in charge for the duration.

- Birthing partner: If your client does not want you to attend, consider training the birthing partner in some simple techniques – they are often grateful to have something to do!

- Frequency and length of reflexology treatments: explain that you will carry out short treatments of about 15 minutes or to meet the client's needs. These can be done when the client lies down to have the baby monitored or you could consider hand reflexology if they want to remain standing.

- Stages of labour: as mentioned, you are most likely to be needed during the first stage of labour. You must make it clear you will not get in the way of the midwife at any point.

- Medical intervention: if at any stage it is considered that the baby needs help to be delivered (forceps, Ventoux, or caesarian), then you will no longer be able to treat the woman.

Reflexology during labour is about being intuitive about what the client needs; if you are only going to have a short time to treat, keep opening and closing moves to a minimum.

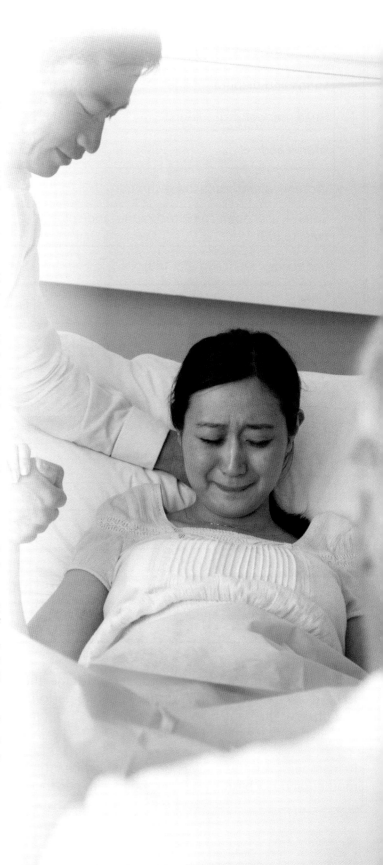

Look at your client and decide if:

1. They are not coping with the frequency and pain of the contractions – if this is the case you need to use reflex points to help calm and regulate breathing.

   Reflex points to concentrate on

Reflex point	Reason
Toe triangle – pituitary, hypothalamus and pineal	Encourages production of endorphins and oxytocin
Solar plexus breathing	Calms and promotes control of breathing
Lungs and diaphragm line	Optimises breathing
Head, neck and shoulders	Aids relaxation
Uterus and cervix	Supports contractions
Adrenal gland – unwind technique	Calms the production of adrenalin
Spine – use 'open spine technique' and spinal twist (p108)	Supports the central nervous system
Endocrine balance (p108-109)	Supports hormone balance
Linking – Uterus, ovaries, adrenals (see Appendix 2)	Eases tension

2. If the contractions are slowing or not dilating the cervix, you should give a deeper treatment aiming at kick starting the contractions again.

   Reflex points to concentrate on

Reflex point	Reason
Toe triangle – pituitary, hypothalamus and pineal	Encourages the production of oxytocin and endorphins
Uterus and cervix	Supports contractions and the dilation of the cervix
Adrenal gland – unwind technique	Calms the production of adrenalin – high levels may slow down contractions
Pelvic area – rub with knuckles	Releases tension in the area
Lumbar spine and coccyx	Releases tension in the area
Spine – use 'open spine technique' and spinal twist (p108)	Supports the central nervous system

Once the labour is heading towards second stage, the woman is usually very inward focused and may not want to have any treatments, but will just let nature perform its miracle. If this is the case, stand out of the way and try and observe the baby being born if you can. It is quite amazing watching a baby being delivered and has never yet failed to make me shed a tear!

Remember: once the baby is born, say how beautiful it is and then it will be time for you to leave and let the mother (and her birthing partner) bond with her/their child.

Common symptoms and lifestyle advice for post natal women

Feeling low

Having a baby can feel like an enormous responsibility and can take up most of the mother's time and energy. It is essential that the mother takes time for herself (reflexology is an excellent way for her to do this!) Motherhood will bring the most joyous days to parents, but can also feel overwhelming at times. If your client is feeling low, remind them that this is normal and suggest they talk about how they are feeling with friends - particularly ones who have had children and therefore will understand and be able to reassure them that it is quite normal to have low periods.

Most women who have had a baby will get offers of help; in the early days, this may be a good time for new mothers to accept help with cooking and cleaning. It is also good if the mother can start to get some gentle exercise every day – even a walk with the pram can help to lift her mood. Also, encourage her to take naps in the days when the baby is sleeping – cleaning can wait!

Baby blues and post-natal depression

It is common for women to suffer from what is commonly called 'baby blues'; this tends to happen between day two and day four after the birth. Baby blues are thought to occur because of the falling hormone levels, mixed with lack of sleep and possibly the overwhelming sense of responsibility for a new tiny life. The mother may feel weepy, anxious, confused and irritated; this is short lived (usually only a few days) and is not classed as post-natal depression, requiring no medical intervention. This is a time when a woman really needs to build in some relaxation time for herself and as a reflexologist you can also:

- Reassure her that it's normal to feel this way.

- Suggest she tries to organise her time and encourage her to leave what can wait.

- Find out if there is a partner or relative who can help with cooking for a few days.

- Encourage her to rest as much as possible.

- Suggest that she keep visitors to a minimum to allow her time to rest when the baby is asleep.

- Listen to her.

If the mother is still feeling depressed after a month, she should see her health visitor or doctor who can assess her. About 10% of women will go on to experience post-natal depression and once diagnosed there should be help from specialised mother-baby units or counsellors.

Common signs of post-natal depression are feeling:

- Anxious

- That they get no pleasure from being a mother

- Possibly suicidal or having thoughts about death

- Guilty and ready to blame herself for everything

- Worthless

- Exhausted and lacking in motivation

- Unable to enjoy herself

- Trapped in her life

- Rejected

- Irritable

- Tearful

- Lonely

If your client expresses these sorts of feelings, you need to ensure that she shares these with a health care worker. If this goes untreated, it can affect the relationship with the baby and may be a problem for a long period.

Some self help ideas:

- Reassure her that there is no such thing as a perfect mum - you learn as you go along.

- Suggest that she:

  - Eats a balanced diet and tries to avoid sugar, chocolate and alcohol; although these are filled with short acting false opiods and may make her feel better in the immediate time, they will only add to the longer term depression.

  - Gets some exercise.

  - Takes some time out for herself.

  - Gets out and about and socialises.

  - Joins a post-natal group or post-natal exercise group.

  - Communicates with her partner, relative or close friend – things often don't feel as bad once you have talked about them.

Reflexology *for* post-natal women

One issue that has arisen has been how hard it can be to get women to come back for treatments once they have had their baby. Yet this is a time when reflexology can be of huge benefit. This is a time when hormone levels drop rapidly and can leave women susceptible to depression. Also, as mentioned, women can feel overwhelmed with the responsibility of looking after such a small, vulnerable new life - and particularly with a first baby, they feel that this tiny new life is totally dictating their lives. If the baby wants feeding, it has to be fed, winded and nappy changed even if you had planned to meet friends.

I saw one client who was post-natal, whose appointment was at 5pm. She looked exhausted and said she had not even managed to have lunch. She could not understand how she had held down an extremely responsible job managing a large team in a city bank and yet one small baby left her unable to even find space to grab a sandwich. This story is not an unusual one. How on earth can they book a reflexology treatment when they don't know what the baby will be demanding?

This is a time when a bit of extra persuasion may be required to try and persuade them to try having a reflexology treatment so they can see it can work - and it is a time when they really need to have some 'me' time. If you have seen the client throughout pregnancy (or even just towards the end of the pregnancy) drop them a congratulations card and include a voucher for a free treatment. If you do not hear from her, after a couple of weeks give her a phone call to see how she is getting on and try and encourage her to have the free treatment.

Generally, this is a time when it easier for the client to have a home visit if you offer these, as she will have everything to hand that she needs. Ideally, suggest she have the treatment when someone is around to look after the baby. She may need to feed the baby whilst having reflexology: this is not a problem (although you will need to make sure she is upright enough to do this), but she can then hand the baby over so she can fully relax. If it is not possible for her to have a treatment when someone else is around, reassure her that it can work extremely well with the baby there. If the baby is asleep when you arrive, then you can start the treatment. If the baby is awake, or wakes during the treatment, ask the mother to just lay the baby on her tummy (baby's tummy onto the mother's tummy), and as long as the baby is not hungry, you will find that the baby calms and will sleep. If the baby is hungry then the mother can feed and wind the baby and then again place the baby on her tummy. You can almost see that as the mother relaxes, this calm energy passes through to the baby – to this date I have never done a treatment with a screaming baby!

You can also finish off by doing a few gentle massage moves on the baby's feet e.g. clockwise rubs over the large intestine area. Remember to say when you meet the baby how beautiful he/she is even if you can't quite see it - mothers always love to hear how beautiful the baby is!

Once the new mum has had a treatment that has worked successfully and has felt the benefit of the reflexology, hopefully they will be back soon for more! Definitely try and get them to book in for their next treatment whilst you are there; this is a group whose days/weeks/ months can just disappear without them having a thought of things they need to plan or book for.

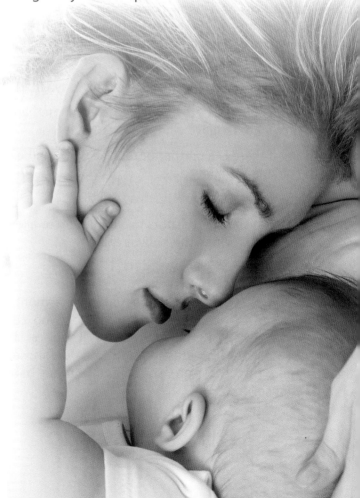

Reflex points to concentrate on for common symptoms:

General post-natal treatment

Reflex point	Reason
Toe triangle (pituitary, hypothalamus and pineal) (p107)	Encourages production of endorphins and oxytocin
Head and brain	Calms any chemical imbalances
Uterus	Helps restore it to its normal state
Lumbar spine	Aids relaxation
Endocrine balance (p108-109)	Helps to rebalance the whole endocrine system
Linking – uterus, ovaries, pituitary (see Appendix 2)	Calms the production of adrenalin

Depression

Reflex point	Reason
Head and brain	Calms any chemical imbalances
Toe triangle (pituitary, hypothalamus and pineal) (p107)	Helps to regulate hormones
Solar plexus	Calms the client's nerves
Spine – use 'open spine technique' and spinal twist (p108)	Promotes the function of the nervous system
Endocrine balance (p108-109)	Supports hormone balance
Linking – Lumbar 5 to hip (see Appendix 2)	Calms the production of adrenalin Relaxes the nervous system

Reflexology to help breast feeding women

Reflex point	Reason
Toe triangle (pituitary, hypothalamus and pineal)	Helps to promote the production of prolactin and oxytocin
Head and brain	Calms any chemical imbalances
Neck and shoulders	Relaxation can help the flow of milk
Solar plexus	Calms the client's nerves
Thoracic nerves	Normalises nerve supply to the breast area
Endocrine balance (p108-109)	Supports hormone balance
Linking – uterus, ovaries, pituitary (see Appendix 2)	Normalises the function of the client's hormones

Research *in maternity reflexology*

This book has provided numerous examples of research into the field of research into maternity reflexology; however, the volume of anecdotal evidence supporting reflexology in maternity is even greater; many women feel they have benefited from having reflexology throughout their pregnancy and gained improvement in their health and general wellbeing. However, this does not provide us with sound evidence that we can use in advertising and marketing. There is now a little scientific evidence that supports the use of reflexology in pregnancy and the postnatal period.

Three recent studies have shown that reflexology in pregnancy:

- Significantly reduced pain during labour (1, 2),

- Reduced the length of the first stage of labour (1, 2).

- Improved quality of sleep in post-natal women (3).

However, most of the other studies looking at reflexology in maternity have not shown significant differences. This is often because the studies have been poorly designed or have not been large enough.

Stress and pregnancy

Another interesting paper by Denise Tiran (4) explores the detrimental effect of stress on pregnancy and states that if "psychological factors (e.g. anxiety) become pronounced, the resulting rise in stress hormones exacerbates physiological changes, leading to complications such as pre-eclampsia, intra-uterine growth retardation, gestational diabetes or pre-term labour".

The paper explains that stressors (physical or psychological) will activate the hypothalamus, which stimulates the autonomic nervous system, which in turn increases levels of catecholamines, adrenalin and noradrenalin. These can all lead to spontaneous abortion during the first trimester or pre-term labour. Therefore, it is important that we do not underestimate how beneficial it can be to have time to relax and de-stress.

The paper then puts forward the argument that complementary therapies (including reflexology) could enhance routine ante-natal care, as they may help to prevent stress induced complications. This is because these therapies increase endorphin and serotonin release, which may add to the mother's ability to cope with the pain by activating the gate pain mechanism.

She concludes by saying that "incorporating touch or relaxation therapies (which includes reflexology) into normal ante-natal care, may be more productive [than current routine care], resulting in women who enter labour in a more relaxed state, consequently normalising the childbearing experience. Relief of physiological disorders of pregnancy, easing of pain in labour, successful breastfeeding and prevention or alleviation of post-natal depression may all be possible, through the use of complementary therapies known to affect stress hormones".

N.B. This paper provides useful information that may be relevant to discuss with your clients, but it does not provide evidence that can be used in advertising or marketing.

References

(1) VALIANI M ET AL (2010) Reviewing the effect of Reflexology on pain and outcomes of the labour of primiparous women. Iranian Journal of Nursing and Midwifery Research. 15(Dec) p302-310

(2) Dolation M ET AL (2011) The effects of Reflexology on Pain Intensity and duration of Labor on Primiparas. Iran Red Crescent Medical Journal. 13(7) p475-479

(3) LI C-Y ET AL (2011) Randomised controlled trial of the effectiveness of using foot reflexology to improve quality of sleep amongst post partum women. Midwifery. 27. p181-186

(4) TIRAN D, CHUMMUN H (2004) Complementary therapies to reduce physiological stress in Pregnancy. Complementary Therapies in Nursing and Midwifery, 10. P162-167. Available online at www.sciencedirect.com

Domestic violence

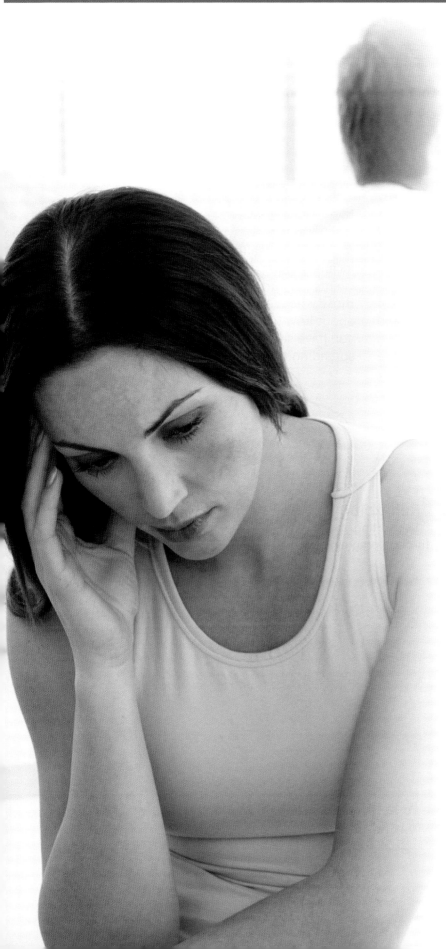

Although it is unlikely that you will see a client who is a victim of domestic violence. If a woman does disclose this to you, it is important that you know where your boundaries lie as a reflexologist. This is not something that you should take on yourself but is a case where the women needs to seek help from her family doctor, social worker, Women's Aid (to arrange a refuge) or the police. You may not refer her unless she gives you permission to do so. It is always best to encourage the woman to seek help.

The AoR constitution states:

- A member shall practise only within the limits of his/ her professional training and competency. No unqualified advice should be given.

- A member who suspects that a client is affected by any condition, medical or otherwise, should advise the client to consult their medical practitioner or Practice Nurse.

A helpful organisation for domestic violence is Women's Aid, who can support the woman and arrange a refuge. They have a website full of information and a 24 hour help line on 0808 2000 247 or 0808 2000 247.

Advertising and marketing reflexology *as a support through pregnancy*

Treating pregnant women is generally a wonderful experience, where you will share plenty of ups and downs with your clients as hormone levels surge. Also, there are many anxieties along the way e.g. concerns about the impending changes in their lives, potential loss of income and extra costs of having a child, fear about the health of the baby, worry about the birth, etc. These factors can leave a woman feeling delighted, anxious, exhilarated, weepy, or exhausted - and sometimes all at once, so make sure you always have a ready supply of tissues.

Reflexology during pregnancy can be of great support to women throughout pregnancy and can help promote general wellbeing. Receiving reflexology during pregnancy allows the client time away from a busy life and gives them a place where they can focus purely on themselves and their growing baby.

Don't underestimate this; make sure you focus on allowing the client time to talk through her fears, anxieties and excitement and also to talk about how she is feeling about welcoming her baby into her life. She may not have any other time that she can focus purely on herself and on her baby.

My experience has been that there are also plenty of women out there who want to do everything they can to ensure a healthy and natural pregnancy - and that includes using reflexology. Approximately 75% of my clients fall into the category of wishing to conceive and those who are pregnant. I have included some tips later about how to start attracting pregnant clients, but once you have seen a few, this is a group who are excellent at spreading the word.

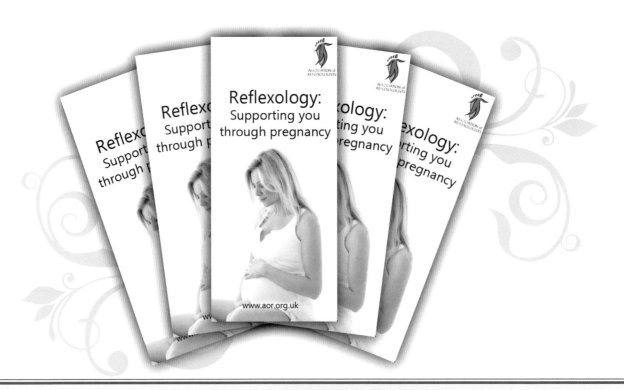

To see a range of products suitable to help you market your practice in this area, visit www.reflexology.org.

Once you have managed to attract your first clients, you will find that they will start to mix with other pregnant women (through ante-natal classes or maybe National Childbirth Trust (NCT) activities) and will start to spread the word about reflexology - hopefully you in particular. It is therefore essential that you give each pregnant client several business cards and ask her to pass them on to friends who may be interested.

Another useful marketing tool is the leaflet produced by the AoR entitled "Reflexology – Supporting you through pregnancy". This leaflet talks about the benefits of receiving reflexology through pregnancy. Again, give each client a few and ask them to hand them out along with your business card.

Starting to attract clients

It is worth thinking about giving talks, so look around your local area and identify where you may be able to offer a talk where you are likely to find your target market, for example:

- NCT ante-natal classes: look on their website (www.nct.org.uk) to find details of your local ante-natal coordinator, make contact with her and ask if you could give a talk and/or leave some leaflets. Incorporate a special offer for any bookings taken in relation to the class and maybe offer the coordinator a free treatment to demonstrate and explain how reflexology can help.

- Toddler workshops: there are likely to be a large number of classes on offer locally for the under 5's e.g. music, drama, gymnastics etc. Although these parents will already have at least one child, many of them will go on to have more. This is also a group of women who will be caught up in the whirlwind of children and could themselves benefit from some 'me' time, so you may attract them as clients as well. Ask to leave some leaflets or give a short talk at the end of a session for those who are interested. Once again it may be a good loss-leader to offer the teacher a free session to get her on board.

- Women's Institute: as an organisation, it appears to be reinventing itself in some areas of the UK; attracting younger women who are your perfect target audience rather than the traditional 'retired jam makers' (not that there is anything wrong with this – but they are likely to be past the age of childbearing. You could still offer to give a general talk on reflexology to the more traditional WIs). Make a call to your local WI and ask about the demographics of the group. Ask whether they would be interested in you giving a talk and demonstration; tailor your talk to the age range of the group.

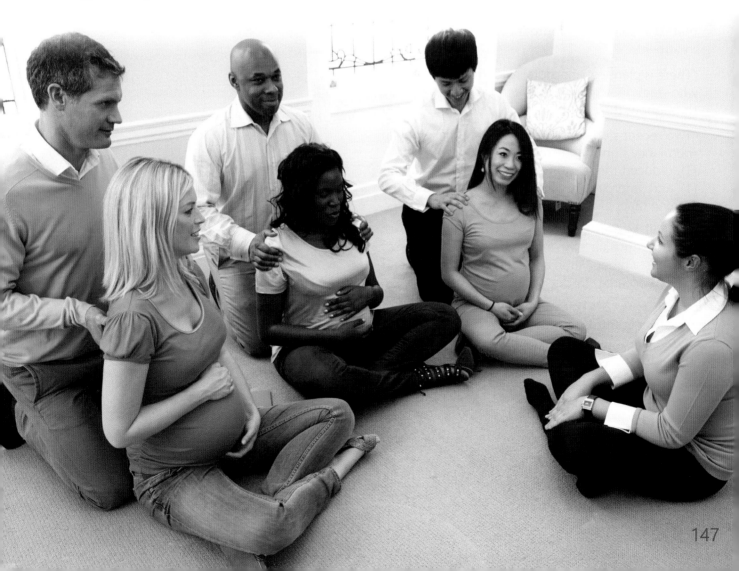

Apart from giving talks, you can also think about local:

- GP Surgeries: many surgeries do not allow promotional material to be put on notice boards as they fear they are held accountable for the service – but it is worth asking.

- Coffee shops /cafés: look around for cafés that are child friendly or have groups of women (perhaps in the lunch hour) and again ask to put leaflets and cards on the notice board. Some may ask for a small payment for you to do this, but you can try it for a couple of months. If you attach a promotional code with a special offer, you will know they have come through the café.

- Editorials: many areas have local magazines and some have dedicated family magazines. Approach them about writing an editorial for which there would be no charge. Alternatively, you could pay for advertising space - but this can be pricey.

When you are considering giving a talk or writing any promotional material, you need to be aware that you must adhere to the Advertising Standards Authority (ASA) regulations. You can use phrases such as:

- "Reflexology aims to optimise the physical and emotional health of pregnant women."

- "Reflexologists work holistically, can provide general lifestyle advice and offer support."

- "Reflexology can be used throughout pregnancy; the reflexologist will take a full history to ensure that it's safe and appropriate to carry out a treatment."

- "There is plenty of anecdotal evidence from women who feel they have benefited from reflexology throughout their pregnancy."

- "Two recent studies have shown that reflexology in pregnancy significantly reduced pain during labour (1), reduced the length of the first stage of labour (1) and improved quality of sleep in post-natal women (2)

(1) VALIANI M ET AL (2010) Reviewing the effect of Reflexology on pain and outcomes of the labour of primiparous women. Iranian Journal of Nursing and Midwifery Research. 15(Dec) p302-310

(2) LI C-Y ET AL (2011) Randomised controlled trial of the effectiveness of using foot reflexology to improve quality of sleep amongst post partum women. Midwifery. 27. p181-186"

N.B. you must quote the references of any research you refer to.

- "Reflexology can be used for general wellbeing or to address other health issues such as sleeping problems as they arise."

- "The therapist will be there to support you through any worries or concerns that you may have."

- "Although there is no evidence that reflexology can induce labour, the general view is that it will help support the body to prepare for labour and promote relaxation at a time when anxiety levels are often high."

I have also put some other information in the post-natal section to give you ideas on how to attract clients back once they have had their baby.

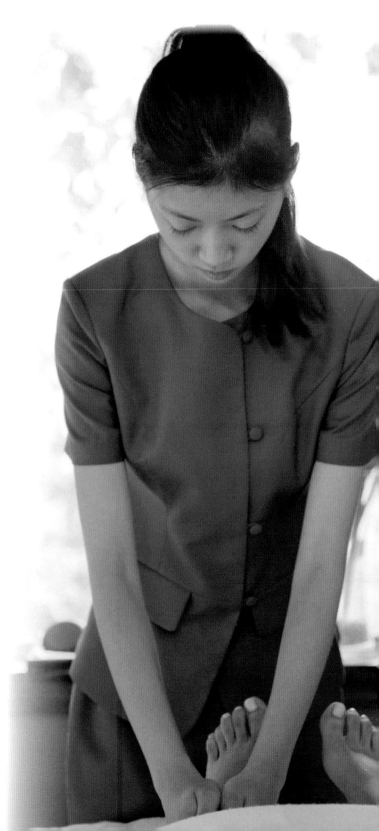

Conclusion

We trust that this guide will prove useful for you in supporting and treating pregnant clients. This is only a guide and don't lose sight of your intuition. It is better to be cautious when treating pregnant women and don't feel afraid to say that you are unsure and/or to seek advice.

Enjoy your treatments of pregnant women. It is a very special time and is a great journey to be able to be with them through all the ups and downs, and then hopefully to be able to share their joy at the end when you finally see mother and baby together.

If this is an area you wish to concentrate on, it is wise to start gaining experience in treating pregnant clients and attend a maternity workshop offered by a fully qualified and experienced tutor, which is a minimum of two days and includes a case study element to further your learning. This will help you gain confidence and work towards becoming experienced in treating pregnant clients. Do be aware that this book is for information and guidance only; if you are unsure, please seek advise from a suitably qualified expert.

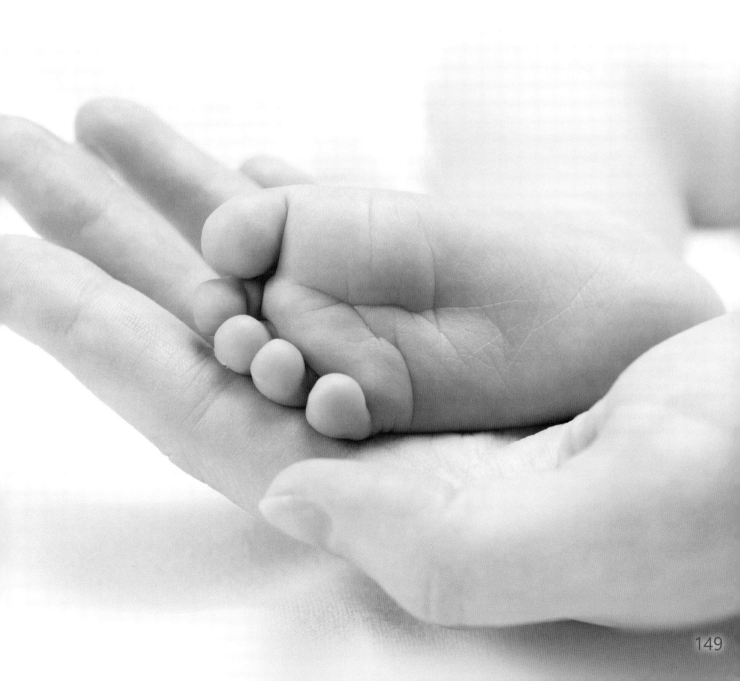

Appendix 1: *maternity reflexology thermometer*

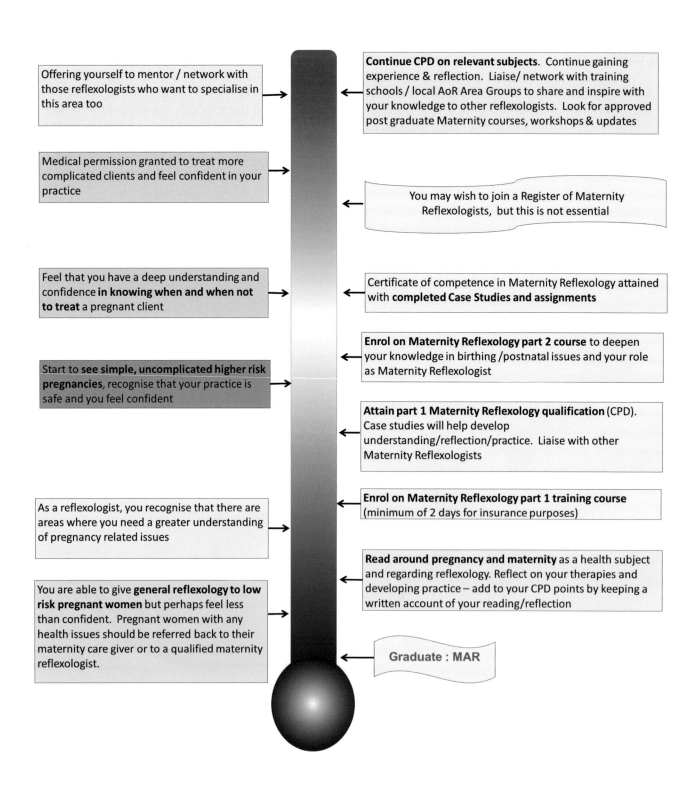

Offering yourself to mentor / network with those reflexologists who want to specialise in this area too

Continue CPD on relevant subjects. Continue gaining experience & reflection. Liaise/ network with training schools / local AoR Area Groups to share and inspire with your knowledge to other reflexologists. Look for approved post graduate Maternity courses, workshops & updates

Medical permission granted to treat more complicated clients and feel confident in your practice

You may wish to join a Register of Maternity Reflexologists, but this is not essential

Feel that you have a deep understanding and confidence **in knowing when and when not to treat** a pregnant client

Certificate of competence in Maternity Reflexology attained with **completed Case Studies and assignments**

Enrol on Maternity Reflexology part 2 course to deepen your knowledge in birthing /postnatal issues and your role as Maternity Reflexologist

Start to **see simple, uncomplicated higher risk pregnancies**, recognise that your practice is safe and you feel confident

Attain part 1 Maternity Reflexology qualification (CPD). Case studies will help develop understanding/reflection/practice. Liaise with other Maternity Reflexologists

As a reflexologist, you recognise that there are areas where you need a greater understanding of pregnancy related issues

Enrol on Maternity Reflexology part 1 training course (minimum of 2 days for insurance purposes)

Read around pregnancy and maternity as a health subject and regarding reflexology. Reflect on your therapies and developing practice – add to your CPD points by keeping a written account of your reading/reflection

You are able to give **general reflexology to low risk pregnant women** but perhaps feel less than confident. Pregnant women with any health issues should be referred back to their maternity care giver or to a qualified maternity reflexologist.

Graduate : MAR

Appendix 2: *linking technique*

Gall bladder to itself

The gall bladder reflex is held with the thumb of one hand, with the middle finger of the other hand holding the point immediately above on the dorsal aspect of the foot.

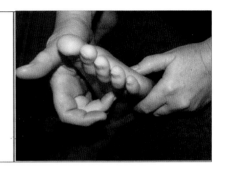

Forebrain to sacrum

One thumb holds the forebrain area on the big toe, the middle finger of the other hand rests on the sacrum reflex.

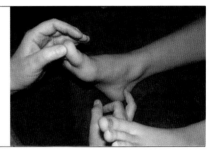

Adrenal to groin

Hold the adrenal reflex with the thumb of one hand. Both middle fingers are then placed on the groin reflexes.

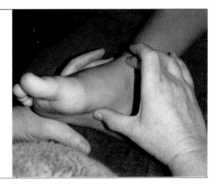

Lumbar 5 to hip

Use one middle finger to locate lumbar 5 on the medial aspect of the foot and the other middle finger to hold the hip reflex.

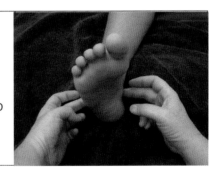

Thymus reflex linked to itself

Place a thumb on the thymus reflex on the plantar aspect of the foot. Use the middle finger of the other hand to hold the point immediately above it on the dorsal aspect of the foot.

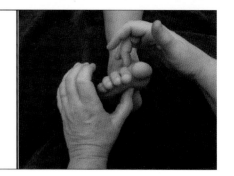

Lung to spine

If there is tension in the lungs at any point (either plantar or dorsal) place one thumb on that point, then take the other thumb directly across to the spinal reflex at the same level.

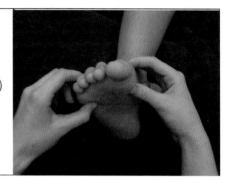

Uterus, ovaries and adrenals

The thumb and third finger of one hand holds the uterus and ovary reflex points, whilst the thumb of the other hand holds the adrenal reflex.

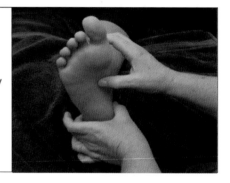

Uterus, ovaries and pituitary

The thumb and third finger of one hand holds the uterus and ovary reflex points, whilst the thumb of the other hand holds the pituitary reflex.

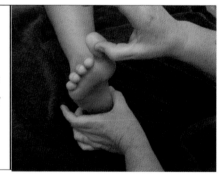